T0280721

CAMBRIDGE LIBRARY COLLECTION

Books of enduring scholarly value

History of Medicine

It is sobering to realise that as recently as the year in which On the Origin of Species was published, learned opinion was that diseases such as typhus and cholera were spread by a ,Äòmiasma,Äô, and suggestions that doctors should wash their hands before examining patients were greeted with mockery by the profession. The Cambridge Library Collection reissues milestone publications in the history of Western medicine as well as studies of other medical traditions. Its coverage ranges from Galen on anatomical procedures to Florence Nightingale,Äôs common-sense advice to nurses, and includes early research into genetics and mental health, colonial reports on tropical diseases, documents on public health and military medicine, and publications on spa culture and medicinal plants.

Observations on Fevers And Other Diseases

Robert Robertson (1742–1829) was a Scottish doctor and surgeon. After completing his medical apprenticeship, Robertson joined the Royal Navy as a surgeon's mate in 1760. In 1768 he was appointed surgeon to the sloop *Diligence,* and served as surgeon on various ships in the West Indies, North America and west Africa until 1783. He was appointed surgeon to the Royal Hospital, Greenwich in 1793. This volume, first published in 1792, contains Robertson's detailed observations of malarial and yellow fever, dysentery and other diseases which he encountered while serving as surgeon in the West Indies. Robertson describes in detail the symptoms and progression of these diseases, his treatments and the outcomes, as recorded in his monthly reviews of the ships' sick lists and many detailed case histories of his patients. This volume provides valuable information concerning the treatment of common diseases and conditions on board late eighteenth-century naval ships.

Observations on Fevers and Other Diseases

Which Occur on Voyages to Africa and the West Indies

Robert Robertson

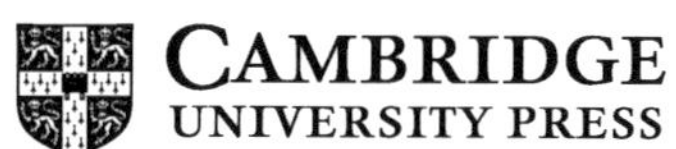

CAMBRIDGE UNIVERSITY PRESS

Cambridge, New York, Melbourne, Madrid, Cape Town, Singapore,
São Paolo, Delhi, Dubai, Tokyo, Mexico City

Published in the United States of America by Cambridge University Press, New York

www.cambridge.org
Information on this title: www.cambridge.org/9781108024341

This edition first published 1792
This digitally printed version 2010

ISBN 978-1-108-02434-1 Paperback

OBSERVATIONS

ON

F E V E R S,

AND OTHER DISEASES,

WHICH OCCUR ON

V O Y A G E S

TO

AFRICA and the WEST INDIES.

By ROBERT ROBERTSON, M.D.

PHYSICIAN TO THE ROYAL HOSPITAL AT GREENWICH.

Deus conamini favebit.

LONDON:

PRINTED FOR JOHN MURRAY, No. 32, FLEET-STREET.

M.DCC.XCII.

ADVERTISEMENT.

AT this Period, when Commerce, eſpecially to Africa and the Weſt Indies, engages ſo much of the public Attention, a new Edition of a Work peculiarly adapted to promote and preſerve the Health of thoſe living in hot Climates, whether on Board or on Shore, cannot fail being highly acceptable, and meeting with ſuitable Encouragement. The original Work appeared many Years ago, under the Title of "A Phyſical Journal, &c." and has been found of very great Utility, as well for the Correctneſs of the Meteorological Remarks, as for the Chaſteneſs of the Medical Obſervations, and Fidelity of the Practice. It is with Pleaſure, therefore, that the Author can look back on his firſt Obſervations, comprehending one grand Source of his univerſal Fever, *Febrile Infection* (though ſubdivided by Writers into many theoretic Species), and find them ſo conſonant to Philoſophy, to Facts, and his univerſally ſucceſsful Treatment of Fevers, that he has no material Error to correct. He therefore ſubmits them to the candid Public, for whoſe Intereſt they were collected; truſting they will generouſly pardon the Style, which, though ſimple, is yet adorned with the brighteſt Ornament—*Truth*. Such as they are, the Author begs leave to inſcribe them to his Friend, JAMES BOGLE FRENCH, Eſq. Chairman of the Committee of Merchants trading to Africa; as a Teſtimony of his Eſteem and Regard.

Royal Hoſpital at Greenwich,
4th April, 1791.

THE

PREFACE

THE following Journals and Obſervations were not curſory remarks made for amuſement in idle or leiſure hours. They are the reſult of an unwearied and cloſe attention to nature and diſeaſes in a diſtant part of the world, and in a climate which yearly proves fatal to many Engliſh ſeamen.

They are offered with all deference to the Publick, as a ſmall addition to what has hitherto been known of thoſe diſeaſes, and as a ſpecimen of a plan for obtaining a further knowledge concerning them, by recommending to Gentlemen of greater abilities and experience, eſpecially Surgeons in the royal navy—the keeping an accurate regiſter of diſeaſes, their ſymptoms, and cure, in the courſe of theſe or other voyages.

Hence, I apprehend publick advantages would accrue. The unexperienced and young Surgeon, ſent to different climates, would, as well as the Pilot who navigates the ſhip, be furniſhed with a guide to avoid errors and miſtakes of moſt dangerous conſequence; and in proceſs of time, a perfect and compleat ſyſtem of the fevers and diſeaſes peculiar to them, would probably be obtained.

It is obvious, that none of the profeſſion can have equal opportunities with the Surgeons of his Majeſty's navy, of knowing the diſeaſes of all the different navigable parts of the world which are incident to ſeamen, and the moſt ſucceſsful manner of treating them, as they are daily viſited by

ſome

ſome of thoſe gentlemen. How much therefore is it to be wiſhed, that they would eſteem it worthy of their trouble, to keep regular journals of the diſeaſes which occur to them every voyage, and of the manner in which they treat them; and that they would communicate them both to the Publick.*

I am very confident what reply many of my Brethren may too juſtly make to this reaſoning : namely, That the little encouragement which we have in the ſervice of the navy, does not merit our attention, or trouble, to promote its benefit. I acknowledge that our encouragement is extremely pitiful; yet, let us not only hope that the time is not far off, when we ſhall poſſeſs a more reſpectable footing in the ſervice, which a joint and ſteady exertion of our abilities will the more readily effect; but conſider, that it becomes us as men, to do every thing in our power in behalf of our fellow creatures; and as Gentlemen, to convince the world, that we make our duty, and the intereſt of his Majeſty's ſervice, our principal ſtudy, notwithſtanding the many hardſhips under which we labour.

I may venture to ſay, that there are ſtill numbers on the liſt of naval Surgeons, who, in abilities, are inferior to none of the profeſſion; and are therefore, every way qualified to extend the knowledge of phyſick. If ſuch Gentlemen would ſet the example before others, of making and communicating ſuch uſeful obſervations to the publick as occur to them from time to time, they would then be convinced, that few of us are ſo deſtitute of underſtanding or emulation, as not to follow it.

I have

* For as it is obſerved by Doctor JAMES LIND, Phyſician of Haſlar hoſpital, the moſt eminent writer on this ſubject, in his Diſſertation on Fevers and Infection, p. 268, of the new edition of his Eſſay on the moſt effectual means of preſerving the Health of Seamen, "Knowledge in phyſick can only be attained by " a ſeries of obſervations, we muſt therefore add to our own experience, that of men who lived before us, " or who practiſe in different places, carefully ſeparating *experienced* truths from *hypotheſes*," &c.

This gentleman, for the good of his Majeſty's ſervice in particular, has wrote ſeveral valuable books, which, taken together, may be eſteemed a Synopſis of the marine practice of phyſick; and alſo contain the neceſſary precepts for preventing ſickneſs on board of his Majeſty's ſhips; but ſurely for reaſons too obvious to mention, it behoves us, at leaſt, to illuſtrate his doctrine.

It is this Dr. LIND whom I have made mention of in the following ſheets.

I have already mentioned the principal reaſon for my publiſhing the following ſheets; but I have likewiſe one great encouragement thereto, which is, that as every attempt to benefit mankind, however ſo far ſhort it may come of the Author's deſign, entitles him, if not to their regard, at leaſt, to their good wiſhes; and I may add without vanity, that if I have failed in obtaining ſo deſireable an end, I have endeavoured at leaſt to deſerve ſucceſs.

As it is an eſtabliſhed rule of the moſt eminent of the antient and modern phyſicians, that he who would practiſe with ſafety and certainty in phyſick, ought to pay particular attention to the ſituation of the country, to its ſoil, and to the water where he does practiſe; as well as to the ſeaſon of the year, the weather, the age and ſex of his patients; and both to his former and preſent way of living; I imagine that it is equally neceſſary to pay due attention to thoſe particulars on board of a ſhip, as nearly as circumſtances there will admit. The following Journal was therefore kept in imitation of the eminent and learned Huxham's *Obſervationes de. aere & morbis epidemicis*, particularly the Monthly Review of the Sick Liſt, though in a far leſs elegant and learned language.

I have only deviated from his plan, where neceſſity obliged me. A barometer upon trial, I found would not anſwer on board, as the motion of the ſhip perpetually agitated the mercury in the tube. Nor could I place an inſtrument on board, ſo as to exactly indicate the quantity of rain which fell in any given time, where the maſts, yards, ſails or ropes, would not have either diminiſhed or added to the real quantity.

The thermometer, which is made by Fahrenheit's ſcale, after the firſt thirty-three days of the firſt voyage, when it was in my own cabbin in the cockpit, always hung in the Captain's cabbin, neither expoſed to the open air, nor the rays of the ſun; conſequently it was in a medium between the air on the lower gun deck, where the men ſlept with the ports down, and that on the upper deck. I have carefully noted the height of the mercury three times a day—Moſt commonly at eight a. m. at noon,

c and

and at eight p. m. at four p m. too, when there was any alteration of its height Oppoſite the hour of the day is the degree of heat; an f follows it, when there was a *fire* in the cabbin; and when the thermometer was expoſed to the rays of the *ſun*, which was only twice, for fear of breaking it, as it is a pretty large one, ſ follows the degree of heat.

The degrees of latitude and longitude are marked after the uſual manner. R in the column of latitude ſignifies that there was no obſervation that day, but was *reckoned* only. L O in the column of longitude, ſignifies a *Lunar* Obſervation; and the degrees under which the two letters are placed, is generally the longitude from London, otherwiſe it is kept either from the laſt departure, or from the place mentioned in the column. In the column of latitudes, in the undermentioned inſtances,* the latitude is not that of the place mentioned, we being nearly oppoſite to it, or ſaw it only.

The moon's age is denoted by figures, 1, 2, &c. p ſignifying the *full*, and m the *change*. The winds are marked with the uſual initials. When f and t occur with two winds, they ſhow that it has blown *from* the firſt *to* the latter, for example, f S t S WbW from ſouth to SWbW. Calm is marked —, very little *, freſh breezes **, gales and ſqualls ***, and very hard gales ****. A tornado is diſtinguiſhed thus ⋇, variable winds by V, ſea breezes by Sb, and land breezes by lb.

Rain is ſpecified by dots. Very light . ſhowers . . heavy . . . very heavy . . . . and dews by ❖ in the ſame column.

The appearances of the atmoſphere are diſtinguiſhed by letters, c. for *clear*, cl. *cloudy*, h. *hazy*, t. *thunder*, and l. for *lightning*.

Throughout the book, a. m. ſignifies *before-noon*, m. ſignifies *noon* and p. m. *afternoon*.

The

* Hiſpaniola, page 38—Lizzard, 44—Cape Coaſt, 52—Beata, 59——Off Cuba 64—Havannah, *ib.* —Scilly, 67—Coaſt of Barbary, 72—Senegal Road, 73—Mayo, 76—Deſeada, 84—Navaſſa, 90—Cape Dona Maria, *ib.*——Off Cape Nicholas, *ib.*—Cape Nicholas Mole, *ib.*—Hiſpaniola, 91—Heniago, *ib.*

The daily Remarks, particularly with refpect to the Sick Lift, are in a feparate column. in the Meteorological Journal, there are ten columns in all which are properly diftinguifhed at the tops thereof.

The practical obfervations on fuch difeafes as occurred during the three different voyages which I made in the Rainbow, together with the method of their having been treated, are briefly fet forth in the Monthly Review; and a more particular account of the remitting Fever and the Dyfentery follow, as they were not only the moft frequent, but the moft dangerous difeafes. The appearance of the urine is feldom noticed becaufe of the difficulty attending that enquiry on board of a fhip.

The Poftfcript contains fome Remarks concerning the prevention of ficknefs from fhore duty on the coaft of Africa; and a Propofition for rendering ficknefs on board of his Majefty's fhips on that coaft lefs fatal than it generally is.

In order that all the obfervations which I had made concerning the remitting fever on the coaft of Africa, might appear together, I thought proper to infert a particular account of the fever which happened there, on board of the Weafel, in the year 1769, previous to the Rainbow's journal, notwithftanding Doctor LIND has been pleafed to give a copy of my journal of that fever, a place in his valuable book, on the difeafes incident to Europeans in hot climates.

I will not pretend to fay that the difeafes which fell under my obfervation upon that coaft, the fhort time which we ftayed each voyage, are all the difeafes that are to be met with there; for a difeafe may happen and be epidemic there one year, as well as in any other part of the world, which may not occur for a number of years following—At leaft I imagine fo.

I have not inferted particular formulæ of medicines, thinking it would have been inconfiftent with my plan to have done it, as I do not deliver a general hiftory of the difeafes, but relate their appearance as they fell under my obfervation, with the manner in which I treated them. The formulæ which

which I uſed, will be thought very ſimple, as they contained no ſuperfluous article to render them elegant or oſtentatious. But let it be conſidered now, that how inelegant ſoever the manner in which I treated my patients may be thought, I could have very eaſily preſented it in a different view to the Publick, if I had choſen to varniſh truth with falſehood. But I chooſe to repreſent facts only. This conſideration, and my motive already mentioned, for offering theſe ſheets to the Publick, will I hope, in ſome meaſure, atone for all the errors and inaccuracies which they contain.

For the ſake of perſpicuity, I have divided the whole into four Parts, and ſubdivided theſe into Chapters and Sections. The firſt part contains an account of the fever which happened in 1769, on board the Weaſel; the ſecond contains the meteorological journal on board of the Rainbow; in the third is contained the Monthly Review of the ſick liſt, and practical obſervations on moſt of the diſeaſes which occurred; and the fourth is taken up with a more particular account of the fever and dyſentery.

CONTENTS.

CONTENTS.

PART I.

An Account of the Remitting Fever which occurred on Board his Majesty's Sloop *Weasel*, on the Coast of *Africa*, in the Year 1769.

CHAPTER I.

Of the Weather and Sick List. Page.

CHAPTER II.

Of the Remitting Fever.

PART II.

The Meteorological Journal and State of the Sick Lift, on board of his Majefty's Ship *Rainbow*, in 1772, 1773, and 1774.

CHAPTER I.

CHAPTER II.

CHAPTER III.

PART III.

The Monthly Review of the Sick Lift.

CHAPTER I.

CHAPTER II.

CHAP-

CHAPTER III.

CHAPTER IV.

Remarks on particular Difeafes.

PART IV.

A particular Account of the Fever and Dyfentery.

CHAPTER I.

Of the Remitting Fever.

CHAPTER II.

Of the Dyfentery.

POSTSCRIPT.

PART

PART I.

An Account of the Remitting Fever, which happened on board of His Majeſty's Sloop Weaſel, on the Coaſt of Africa, in the Year 1769.

CHAPTER I.

OF THE WEATHER AND SICK LIST.

SECTION I.

An Abſtract of the Weather from the Ship's Log Book, with Remarks on the Sick Liſt, between the 13th of June and the 8th of September 1769.

PREVIOUS to the account of the remitting fever, I beg leave to inſert an abſtract of the weather from the ſhip's log book, with the daily ſtate of the ſick liſt, which I hope will not be deemed an improper introduction, as it will appear from thence how far the weather can be ſaid to have been acceſſory to the riſe of this fever.

In the following abſtract the ſame ſignatures are made uſe of as in the Rainbow's meteorological journal.

Year, Months, and Days.	Latitude or different parts.	Longitude made.	Winds.	Rain or Dew	Appearances of the Atmosphere.	REMARKS, AND STATE OF THE SICK LIST
1769 Junii 13 Die Martis	Turning down the channel		fNNW tWSW *	.	a. m. c.	Sailed a. m. from Plymouth found with three in the list. —one fever, one intermittent, and one cold.
14	49° 20″ R.	From the Lizzard 00° 43″W	fSWBS tNNW * *	.	a.m. cl. p.m. c.	One fever from cold added to the list ; four in it.
15	47° 37 R.	02° 08″W	fNWBN t W *	.	a. m. c. p.m. cl.	One contusion added to the list; five in it.
16	45° 19″	03° 41″W	fW tNW **		cl.	The cold of the thirteenth well; four in the list
17	43° 45″ R.	04° 20″W	fNWBN tWBN *		cl.	One wound added to the list ; five in it.
18	41° 30″	11° 24″W from London.	fNWBW tNE **		cl.	One headach added to the list; six in it.
19	39° 45″	12° 02″W	NE *		cl.	Yesterday's headach well ; five in the list
20	37° 50″	12° 48″W	f NE t NNE **		a. m. c. p.m. cl.	The fever of the fourteenth, and the contusion of the fifteenth well ; three in the list.
21	35° 47″	13° 34″W	f NNE t N		c.	No alteration in this day's list.
22	34° 08″	from London. 14° 14″W	NNE N		m. cl.	Three in the list.
23	33° 03″	15° 27″W	NNE N *		c.	No alteration in the list.
24	31° 49″ Madeira		fNBE t NE *		a. m. c. p.m. cl.	The intermittent of the thirteenth well; two in the list.
25	29° 50″		NBE N *		cl.	One sore throat, and one with eruptions added to the list ; four in it.
26	28° 30″ St. Cruze Teneriff		V *		cl.	The intermittent, returned well the 24th, relapsed; five in the list.
27			V *		c.	No alteration in the list.
28			f NE t NW *		c.	One sore throat added to the list; six in it. The weather very warm.

Year, Months, and Days.	Latitude or different Parts.	Longitude made.	Winds.	Rain or Dew.	Appearances of the Atmosphere.	REMARKS, AND STATE OF THE SICK LIST.
Junii 29			V **		m. cl.	The one added the 25th with eruptions well; five in the lift.
30			f NW t NE *		c.	One ftrain added to the lift; fix in it—one bad fever, one intermittent, one wound, two fore throats, and one ftrain.
Julii 1 Die Saturni			V & —		c.	The fore throat of the 28th ult. well, and the other fore throat is a venereal; four in the lift.
2			NE NNW *		cl.	The wound of the 17th, and the ftrain of the 30th ult. are well
3			V *		c.	One ftrain, and one contufion added to the lift; four in it.
4			V *		c.	Yefterday's contufion well, and one tumor added to the lift.
5			NE SE *		c.	One feverifh complaint added to the lift; five in it.
6			V *		c.	No alteration in the lift.
7			V *		h. & cl.	The ftrain of the 3d, the tumor of the 4th, and the fever of the 5th well; two in the lift.
8			V *		a.m. cl. p. m. c.	The fever of the 13th ult. died; and one contufion added to the lift; two in it.
9			V		a. m. c p.m. cl.	No alteration in the lift, p. m. very fultry.
10			V *		c.	The lift the fame.
11	Turning up to windward		f ESE t NE *		m. cl.	No alteration in the lift. Sailed to day.
12	28° 36″		f NNE t ENE **		cl.	Two in the lift.
13	Porto Orotavia Teneriff		V *		a. m. c. p.m. cl.	One naufea added to the lift; three in it. Seven p. m. anchored in the road which is quite open.
14			V *		cl.	The contufion of the 8th, and yefterday's complaint well, and one naufea added to the lift; two in it.
15			V *		cl.	One headach added to the lift; three in it.

Year, Months, and Days.	Latitude or different parts.	Longitude made.	Winds.	Rain and Dew.	Appearance of the Atmosphere.	REMARKS, AND STATE OF THE SICK LIST.
16			NE *		cl.	One contusion added to the list ; four in it.
17	27° 49″		f NNE t EBS *		p. m. c.	One nausea added to the list ; five in it. Sailed from Teneriff.
18	25° 01″		f EBN t EBS ***		a m. c. p.m. cl.	Yesterday's complaint a fever, and one nausea added to the list ; six in it.
19	21° 49″		ENE E ***		m. cl.	Yesterday's nausea well ; five in the list.
20	19° 08″	16° 57″	ENE WBN***		c.	The contusion of the 16th well, and one lumbago added to the list ; five in it.
21	17° 31″	From London 16° 18″	V ***		c.	The headach of the 15th well ; and yesterday's lumbago.
22	16° 13″ Barbary Coast.		V *		c.	The nausea of the 14th well ; and one strain added to the list ; three in it.
23	15° 54″ Senegal Road.		NBE and NBW *		c.	The nausea of the 17th well, two in the list. Anchor'd p. m. and sent a boat up to the fort.
24			NBE and NBW **		c.	Two in the list.
25	15° 33″		V *		a. m. c. p. m. h. & cl.	No alteration in the list, p. m. sailed.
26	15° 05″		V *		p m. cl.	Two in the list.
27	Off Cape De Verde		WNW *		h. & cl.	No alteration in the list.
28	Off Gambia River		NNW *		h. & cl	One contusion and one tumor added to the list ; four in it.
29			NNW *		h. & cl.	No alteration in the list. Spoke h. m. Sloop Hound and got a man out of her to pilot us up the river—he had a very sickly complexion. P. m. Standing in to wards the river.
30	Gambia River		V **	. . . . ❖	a. m. h. & cl.	The Hound's man added to the list with a fever, five in the list. Getting up the river a. m. and anchored p. m.
31			V *	. . . . ❖	a. m. & p.m. cl. & h.	No alteration in the list. Men sent a shore to cut wood. The river is very shallow, and the land on each side of

Year, Months, and Days.	Latitude or different parts.	Longitude made.	Winds.	Rain or Dew.	Appearances of the Atmosphere.	REMARKS, AND STATE OF THE SICK LIST.
						of it, which is covered with thick woods, is very low, with a thick haze constantly over it and the iver. Our men have been exposed to the rains. Two intermittents—the hound's man is one—one strain, one contusion, and one tumor.
Augusti Die Martis 1			V *	❖	cl. & h.	The contusion of the 28th well; four in the list. Sailed up the river and run a ground near Fort James; which occasioned the men's being very much fatigued in the heat of the sun. A very sultry day.
2			and V	❖	cl. & h.	Two feverish complaints added to the list; six in it. Got the ship off and anchored, after much trouble in the sun. The Fort—and we were nearly opposite to it—is on a small island seven leagues up the river; which is about six miles broad there, and shallow. On the Barra side where the watering place is, it is very swampy and covered with trees, and shrubs. The water was thickish but had no bad taste. The men were obliged to swim the casks off, as a boat could not get near the shore. A continual haze notwithstanding the sun shines.
3			— and V	❖	cl. & h	One of yesterday's fevers is an intermittent Six in the list.
4			V ⁂	. . . . ❖	cl.t.& l.	No alteration in the list. The two last added intermittents are very ill. The men are employed in watering the ship.
5			SW —	. . . . ❖	cl.	No alteration in the list. Disagreeable weather.
6			Wly —	❖	cl.	The tumor of the 28th ult. well. Five in the list.
7			V ⁂	. . . . ❖	cl.t & l.	One of the feverish of the 2d. well. Most of the officers and gentlemen have been a shore—which was all a marsh—a shooting. Four in the list.
8	Sailing down the river		V and —	❖	cl.t.& l.	Five with feverish, two with purging complaints, and one with eruptions, added to the list; twelve in it. Sailing and anchoring now and then.
9	13° 40″ Sailing down the river		V *	. . ❖	cl.	One with a purging added to the list; thirteen in it.
10	13° 41″	15° 49″ from London W	V ⁂	. . . . ❖	cl.t.&.l	No alteration in the list. Got out of the river. Very disagreeable weather.

Year, Months, and Days.	Latitude or different parts.	Longitude made.	Winds.	Rain or Dew.	Appearances of the Atmoſphere.	REMARKS, AND STATE OF THE SICK LIST.
11	13° 55″ R	16° 30″ W	V *	.. ❖	cl. & h.	One of the fluxes of the 8th, and one of the fevers, with the purging of the 9th well; four ſlight fevers added to the liſt; fourteen in it.
12	14° 06″ R	17° 00″ W	V *	.. ❖	cl. & h	One of the bad intermittents of the 2d. well; p. m. one ſlight fever added to the liſt; fourteen in it. The fevers are ſlight though of the remitting kind.
13	12° 54″	17° 04″ W	V **	.... ❖	cl. & h	Two of the fevers of the 11th well, and one purging complaint added to-day; thirteen in the liſt. Sultry diſagreeable weather.
14	11° 30″	17° 34″ W	ſNWBW t NNE **	.. ❖	cl. & h.	The old intermittent, the Hound's man, one of the ſlight fevers of the 8th, and the one with eruptions well; ſix fevers added to the liſt,
15	10° 47″ R	17° 45″ W	SBW **	... ❖	cl & h.	One fever added to the liſt; ſixteen in it. Very diſagreeable weather.
16	10° 18″ R	17° 20 W	SW **	. ❖	cl. & h.	Two fevers of the 8th one of the 11th, one of the 12th and the purging of the 13th well; four fevers added to the liſt. Thoſe added the 14th and ſince are bad remittents. Fifteen in the liſt.
17	09° 33″	16° 46″ W	SW **	.... ❖	cl. & h.	One of yeſterday's fevers well; two fevers, one diarrhæa, and one headach added to the liſt; eighteen in it.
18	08° 38″ R	15° 55″ W	V *	.... ❖	cl.	One of the fevers of the 8th, one of the 11th, and yeſterday's headach well; ſeven fevers added to the liſt, and one who was in it before become feveriſh; twenty two in the liſt. Moſt of them bad remittents.
19	08° 05″	14° 31″ W	SW *	❖	cl.	The diarrhœa, and one of the fevers of the 17th well, two fevers, one diarrhœa and the fever of the 8th returned well yeſterday relapſed; twenty four in the liſt. A few of the fevers are attended with a purging.
20	07° 26″	12° 04″ W	SW *		c.	The ſlight fever of the 11th, returned well 16th, relapſed two fevers, and two with a diarrhæa added to the liſt; twenty-nine in it Moſtly fevers and very bad ſymptoms amongſt them.
21	06° 30″	10° 37″ W	SW *	. ❖	cl. & h.	P M. one of the fevers of the 14th died. Very bad ſymptoms amongſt the fevers. Rather cold to-day. Twenty-eight in the liſt.
22	Off Cape monſerado		SW *	❖	cl.	Three fevers, and one hypochondriack added to the liſt; thirty two in it.
23	05° 33″ R	09° 38″ W	SW *		cl.	No alteration in the liſt. Very bad ſymptoms ſtill with the fevers.

Year, Months, and Days.	Latitude or different parts.	Longitude made.	Winds.	Rain or Dew.	Appearances of the Atmosphere.	REMARKS, AND STATE OF THE SICK LIST.
24	05° 13″	09° 29″ W	SW *		c.	One of the fevers of the 16th—a boy—died; and the hypochondriack well; four fevers added to the list; thirty four in it. One seized with the fever to-day by contagion.
25	04° 07″	08° 36″ W	SW *		cl.	One fever added to the list; thirty five in it; and mostly very bad fevers.
26	04° 11″	07° 08″ W	SW **		cl.	One of the fevers of the 17th died. There are very few of the people who are not ailing more or less; though thirty four only are in the list.
27	04° 34″	06° 20″ W	SW *	❖	h.	Two fevers died, one added the 18th, and the other the 20th; thirty two in the list. The ship is frequently washed with vinegar, and was smoaked to day. Very dangerous symptoms amongst the sick.
28	05° 06″	06° 08″ W from London.	SWBW *	❖	h.	Two fevers died, one of them was added the 18th, and the other the 20th—Their deaths happen unexpectedly—thirty in the list.
29	05° 08″	05° 37″ W	V *	❖	h.	One fever of the 14th, one of the 16th, and two of the 24th well; twenty six in the list.
30	04° 57″	04° 51″ W	V *	❖	h.	One fever who was added the 18th died; twenty five in the list.
31	04° 41″	04° 06″ W	V *	❖	h.	One fever who was added the 24th died; and one fever added to the list.
Die Veneris Sept. 1	04° 55″	03° 14″ W	V *	· ❖ ·	h.	One fever who was added 18th died; two fevers of the 20th, two of the 24th, one of the 22d, and one of the 28th, ult. all well; one fever—relapsed—added to the list; nineteen in it. Mostly fevers, and very bad symptoms yet.
2	05° 17″	03° 08″ W	WSW —		a. m. c. p. m. h.	The yesterday's relapse well, and two fevers added to the list—one is a relapse—twenty in it. Anchor'd several times to-day.
3	05° 22″		V & —		a. m. c. p. m. h.	One of yesterday's fevers well; nineteen in the list. Turning up to Winnebah. Anchor'd several times to-day again.
4	Winnebah road		V *		c.	No alteration in the list. Anchor'd off Winnebah.
5			SW		cl.	Nineteen in the list The worst of the fevers geting better. The rains have been over here some time, and the people ashore all well.

Year, Months, and Days.	Latitude or different parts.	Longitude made.	Winds.	Rain or Dew.	Appearances of the Atmosphere.	REMARKS, AND STATE OF THE SICK LIST.
6.			SW & —		h.	Two fevers of the 19th, and the diarrhœa, ult. well; ſixteen in the liſt.
7			V *		cl. & h.	Sixteen in the liſt. Watering the ſhip here.
8			V *	. .	cl. & h.	A diarrhœa added to the liſt; ſeventeen in it. We had no more fevers added to the liſt afterwards.

SECTION II.

A Review of the Sick Liſt, from the 13th June until the Commencement of the Fever, together with ſeveral Practical Caſes.

OUR Complaints from the 13th of June to the end of the month were one bad fever; one intermittent, who got well and relapſed; two colds with feveriſh complaints; two ſore throats---one of them was veneral; one with eruptions; one wound; one contuſion; and one ſtrain.

None of theſe complaints required any particular treatment, except the bad fever, which ſhall be deſcribed in the next month.

We continued very healthy all the month of July; having but few complaints, and none of them dangerous but the Hound's man who was added in the latter end of the month. They were one bad intermittent; three ſlight fevers; two nauſeas; one head ach; one lumbago; four contuſions; two ſtrains; and two abſceſſes.

The ſlight fevers, nauſeæ, and the head ach, were removed by gentle evacuations, ſaline draughts with antimonials, elix. vitriol, and a proper regimen.* The other complaints—except the Hound's man—required no particular method of treatment; but the bad fever of laſt month died the 8th of July, an account of which I beg leave to inſert. John Lee, marine, aged about 30 years, was taking bark for an intermittent, of which he was recovering, when he was ſeized the 13th of June, after having got cold, with general tremors, convulſions, loſs of ſpeech, and cold extremities. His pulſe was quite languid and irregular. Volatiles were uſed, and large bliſters applied to his back, and ankles. Second day, the convulſions were abated, but the tremors continued; and he was coſtive.

* The diet allowed the Sick is mentioned, Part II. ch. 1. ſect. 5.

coſtive. A clyſter was adminiſtered, and a large ſpoonful of a cordial julap preſcribed every hour. 3d, His pulſe was firmer, and he ſpoke pretty ſenſibly; but his tongue was very foul. His bliſters were renewed; his medicines continued; and he was allowed wine. 4th, His tongue was browniſh. Fifteen grains of bark were added to every doſe of the julap. 5th, 6th and 7th, His tongue was much cleaner, but the coma continued. His medicines were repeated, with wine, and the bliſters renewed. 8th and 9th, He was much better, and continued the bark and julap every two hours with his wine. 10th, From drinking beer the preceding afternoon an acceſſion of fever came on; attended with a quick ſmall pulſe, a dry hot ſkin, a parched tongue and a fluſhed countenance: his right ſide was in ſome meaſure paralytick and he had convulſive twitches at times. The nervous medicines, wine, and bliſters were preſcribed. 11th, The fever remitted imperfectly, and the convulſions went off, but the coma continued. I ſtill continued his medicines and wine. 12th, He was cool, but extremely weak. 13th, He was hot, and no way better. 14th, 15th, 16th, 17th and 18th, He was conſiderably better, and continued his medicines with wine. 19th, *p. m.* He became much worſe, but ſtill took his medicines. 20th and 21ſt, He was much weaker; the tremors returned; his tongue was black; and his pulſe quick, and very ſmall. On the 22d, the tremors were conſtant, and his pulſe was very irregular. The muſk julap and wine were continued, and freſh bliſters applied. 23d, 24th and 25th, Deglution became difficult, and his pulſe vermicular, with a ſubſultus tendinum, and continual tremors. His medicines and bliſters were continued, but he died at midnight of the 25th.

From the 1ſt of Auguſt to the 14th, one bad intermittent; eleven ſlight fevers; four diarrhœas, and one with eruptions complained.

The ſlight fevers were of the remitting kind, but very mild; and were all carried off by gentle emetics, purges, the ſaline draughts with antimonials, elixir of vitriol, and proper diet. One of them had an acute pain in his ſide, for which I took away a little blood; and he recovered very well. Some of them were ſeized with the bad fever afterwards, of which ſeveral of them died.

The diarrhœa were likewiſe cured by moderate evacuations and a ſuitable diet.

Before we proceed further, I ſhall relate the two bad intermittent caſes; and I call them intermittents becauſe there was a total ceſſation of the fever and ſymptoms between the paroxyſms, notwithſtanding they were of the tertian kind.

David Clency, ſeaman, aged about 38 years, pretty ſtout, of a very ſickly complexion, complained the 31ſt of July, the day after he came from the Hound, that he was ſeized with a chillineſs, which was ſucceeded by a violent head ach, a ſickneſs at ſtomach, with a reaching to puke, ſevere pains in all his bones, particularly in his loins, and of great thirſt. His pulſe was quick, but not ſtrong; his ſkin very hot and dry, and his tongue was dry and white. I preſcribed the tartar emetic in ſmall quantities every half hour until it puked

 him;

him; and in two hours afterwards I ordered him a ſaline draught with thirty drops of the eſſen. antimon. and acidulated ſage tea for his drink.

2d, The paroxyſm ended in a profuſe perſpiration towards morning; after which he continued perfectly cool and eaſy until 6 *p. m.*—the ſame time of the former fits commencing—when another paroxyſm returned, which was leſs violent than the preceding one, and continued a ſhort time. A doſe of the Sal. cath. amar. was preſcribed, and the ſaline draught as before, during the fit, with drink which was acidulated with lime juice.

3d, He had a ſhort paroxyſm in the night; was free of fever; but complained of weakneſs in his loins; and want of appetite. At 7 *p. m.* a paroxyſm commenced with rigours, which laſted an hour, and ended in the uſual manner. During the fit he complained of great pain and ſtricture over his eyes. The medicine preſcribed the preceding night was repeated every three hours; with tinct. theb. for his headach, which it relieved.

4th, He was very cool and eaſy; but at the uſual time *p. m.* a mild paroxyſm commenced, which did not continue long. His medicines and drink were repeated.

5th, He complained of weakneſs and a little headach; but never had another paroxyſm. Half a drachm of the bark was preſcribed every two hours. Afterwards he took a drachm of it every two hours until he recovered on the 15th of his illneſs.

Serjeant Gilleſpy, about 27 years of age, who had had a ſlight fever the preceding month, was ſeized the 1ſt of Auguſt with chillineſs and rigours, which were ſucceded by the ſame complaints as Clency's were, only in a more violent degree, with an acute pain in his right ſide. But after the paroxyſm went off he had neither fever nor pain. He complained the 2d, when both the emetick and purge were preſcribed; and the ſaline mixture with eſſ. antimon. at night. At 7 *p. m.* the paroxyſm returned. 3d, The paroxyſm went off in the night and he was quite cool and eaſy. I ordered him half a drachm of the bark every two hours during the intermiſſion. 4th, He had a very ſhort, and mild paroxyſm in the night. His bark was repeated every hour. He had no return of his fever afterwards; but continued taking bark until the 12th. When he returned to duty.

Such was the ſtate of our ſick liſt from the time of our leaving England until the 14th of Auguſt, when the fatal remittent made its appearance. A boy of 13 years of age was the firſt taken ill with it on the 12th, but did not complain before the 14th. The complaints of thoſe who were firſt ſeized with the bad remittent ſeemed to differ very little at firſt from thoſe of the preceding ſlight remittent: but was much alarmed when I found, that inſtead of perfect remiſſions neither their fever or other complaints went off; that they had a continual pain in their loins, which was greatly encreaſed during the paroxyſm; that they

had

had a burning heat in the palms of their hands, and ſoles of their feet, with great thirſt; and that they were exceedingly dejected during the imperfect remiſſion. This obſervation made me the more uneaſy becauſe the ſick liſt was hourly encreaſing with ſimilar complaints. I therefore call this a remitting fever, becauſe there never was an entire ceſſation thereof, or of the ſymptoms, from its commencement until a favourable criſis or death happened.

The following obſervations concerning this fever were exactly copied from the minutes which I made frequently in the day when viſiting the ſick, and immediately after reduced, nearly, into the ſame order as they now appear in Doctor Lind's book * on hot climates—and upon the moſt accurate review of my minutes, I have been able to add very little to that account of the fever.

Some had the fever in a mild, and others in a malignant form, comparatively ſpeaking; I ſhall therefore firſt relate the daily ſymptoms which appeared amongſt them who had it in the mildeſt form; ſecondly, relate the ſymptoms which daily occured amongſt thoſe who had it in a malignant form; thirdly, make ſome remarks upon the ſymptoms and the days which proved critical; fourthly, inſert the manner in which I treated them; fifthly, add a few caſes; and laſtly, conclude this firſt part of the work with a few obſervations concerning the cauſe of the fevers having prevailed on board.

CHAPTER II.

OF THE REMITTING FEVER.

SECTION I.

The Fever deſcribed in its mildeſt Form.

1ſt Day. THEY who had the remitting fever in its mildeſt form, complained of a headach, ſickneſs at their ſtomachs, thirſt, great uneaſineſs, with ſevere pains, eſpecially in their backs and loins. Their pulſes were ſmall and quick; and though ſome of their ſkins were hotter and dryer than in health, moſt of them were chilly and hot alternately.

Their complaints were eaſier in the morning; but towards night there was always an exacerbation of them throughout the fever.

2d, They

* See the Note, page 58 of the ſecond edition

2d, They were more lively, and their complaints relieved; but their pulſes were ſoft and weaker than in a natural ſtate; and they had no appetite.

3d, Their ſymptoms became more violent, with giddineſs; inſatiable thirſt; foul tongues, which trembled when they put them out; they had no ſenſation of taſte; and their ſpeech was weak and faultering. At night they had a moiſture on their ſkins.

4th, They were much weaker; and towards night they were very hot and reſtleſs. Numbers ſweated profuſely, which did not refreſh them.

5th, A few had been delirious in the night; and were much diſturbed in their ſleep with frightful dreams and notions. Their weakneſs increaſed. Hitherto they were not confined to bed in the day time.

6th, They were more reſtleſs from anxiety and a delirium. Their tongues were browniſh, dry and chapt.

7th, Towards night they complained much more. The delirium, watching, univerſal uneaſineſs, and their thirſt, being all increaſed.

8th, They had a very bad night; and complained much more of their backs, loins, and giddineſs. *P. m.* their pulſes were very irregular, and generally weaker than in a natural ſtate, the three preceding days; and their tongues were become blackiſh and chopped.

9th, The remiſſion was more diſtinct in the day than hitherto; but an exacerbation of the fever and ſymptoms returned at night.

After this day there was a perfect remiſſion of the fever in the day time; though they became feveriſh towards night until the 17th; and in one caſe the fever continued to return until the 21ſt.

The criſis of the fever was a gentle purging with an equable and moderate perſpiration.

SECTION II.

Deſcription of the Fever in its malignant Form.

1ſt Day, THEY who had the fever in its malignant form, beſides thoſe ſymptoms which they had in common with the other patients —though in a more violent degree—were ſeized with ſome other of the following; deſpondency, great laſſitude, proſtration of ſtrength and ſpirits, anxiety, giddineſs, violent reachings, ſevere gripings and purgings, coſtiveneſs, cough, a violent pain and ſtricture over the eyes, a pain in the ſide, a quick hard pulſe, and a dry and white tongue.

2d, They only who had been both vomited and purged, ſeemed to be a very little better, but had no appetite.

3d, Some

3d, Some had a ſlight remiſſion until the evening approached; their countenances in the mean time were much fluſhed.

4th, Great inquietude, anxiety, frightful dreams, and idle notions, prevented them from ſleep. When a remiſſion happened, it not laſt above three hours. They ſeemed then a little cooler, but their thirſt was not abated; beſides there was a burning heat in the palms of their hands, and ſoles of their feet, and their memories began to fail. The tongues of ſome were white and foul, though in general they were dry and chapped, and they complained of a bad taſte in their mouths. They who were coſtive at the beginning continued ſo; but ſeveral were ſeized with bilious vomitings, and purgings.

5th, Several were delirious in the night; and others exceedingly reſtleſs and deſirous to get out of bed. Some of their tongues were black, and their teeth covered with ſordes; and the cough was much more urgent.

6th, In the morning a few had a ſmall remiſſion, though they all had a very bad night. The pains of their backs and loins; their giddineſs, with a ſevere pain at the bottoms of the orbits, were exceedingly troubleſome. The coſtiveneſs was more obſtinate, and all the other complaints increaſed in violence.

7th, The delirium was more general. Some of their countenances were quite yellow, and others looked wild. A ſcalding of the urine—not from bliſters—rough, brown tongues, a ſmacking of the lips, were frequent for ſome days before, and the vomiting and looſe fetid ſtools were more general. Their pulſes were irregular.

8th, A few after violent vomitings and purgings which both ſtained like an infuſion of ſaffron, broke out in purple blotches like the ſtinging of nettles, particularly about the face and neck, which ſoon diſappeared again.—While they remained out on the ſkin they thought themſelves better.—In one patient the parotid gland began to ſuppurate. The tongues of ſome were black and their teeth cruſted over with black ſordes; but of others, they were browniſh, dry, and much chapped. The delirium, a ſtupor, convulſive tremors, and catchings, twitchings of the tendons, hiccup, deep ſighs, pain and oppreſſion about the præcordia, ſwelling of the hypochondria, cold ſweats, an involuntary diſcharge of the urine and fæces, and a muttering or murmuring inarticulately, were frequent. Their pulſes were quite irregular.

9th, The bad ſymptoms continued. One who had the purple blotches, likewiſe had an hæmorrhage from the noſe and mouth at times, which tinged his linen yellow, as did his urine too, which was bloody.

10th, A few had a very ſlight remiſſion.

11th, The dangerous ſymptoms prevailed, with a coma, cold clammy ſweats, and extreme weakneſs. In one patient a large ecchymoſis-like ſwelling appeared upon the right ſide of the neck and face a little before his death, which immediately after it, became black.

12th, There were no favourable appearances. They continued to lie on their backs as they had done for ſome days.

13th, Their countenances became more generally yellow; and a purging, without gripes, came on. Theſe patients were much relieved, never being afterwards ſo hot and reſtleſs towards night; and one had an equable and gentle perſpiration broke out over him. An eruption appeared about ſome of their mouths. But the dangerous ſymptoms continued in other caſes, with frequent faintings in one patient.

14th, Gripes when at ſtool now attended their purging; and though they were very weak their fever and other complaints were much leſs. The dangerous ſymptoms prevailed ſtill amongſt ſome, with a ſubſultus tendinum; a dozing with the eyes half, and the mouth wide open; and a cadaverous ſmell. Their ſkins were very diſagreeable to the touch, and from feeling the pulſe, an uneaſy ſenſation was impreſſed on the fingers, which continued for ſome time after.

15th, The bad ſymptoms continued; the parotis was opened; and the fluxed patients with the yellow countenances were better: one of whom had the piles.

16th, Though extremely weak they were all better except one man, who had a ghoſtly countenance, and all the dangerous ſymptoms.

17th, The bad caſe was not better, but all the reſt were.

18th, The dangerous caſe fell into a ſound ſleep, and an equable perſpiration broke out over him, which fortunately proved a favourable criſis, and the reſt continued to recover

SECTION. III.

Remarks on the Fever in both its Forms.

WITH reſpect to the following ſymptoms it is to be underſtood, that ſeveral of them perhaps often occurred in one patient.

They who were coſtive when they firſt complained, and continued ſo, all died. The bilious vomitings and ſtools which ſtained like an infuſion of ſaffron were mortal. A hæmorrhage at the noſe and mouth, and bloody urine, all of which tinged yellow, were mortal. The purple blotches which roſe above the ſkin like the ſtinging of nettles, were mortal. An intenſe coma was mortal. An ecchymoſis-like ſwelling upon the face and neck immediately preceded death. One who was taken ill at firſt with a pain in the ſide died. A brown rough

rough tongue and mouth, with a ſmacking of the lips, was mortal. A wildneſs of the countenance was mortal—One perſon who had this ſymptom was very coſtive too, and never ſeemed to be in imminent danger, nor was ever confined to his bed, though he died on the eighth day. A deſpondency, and dread of dying were mortal. A general coldneſs with clammy ſweats, and muttering or murmuring inarticulately, immediately preceded death. A ſyncope or deliquium was mortal.

A cough proved fatal in two caſes out of three; and the third was the remarkable caſe which was dangerous until the eighteenth day. An involuntary diſcharge of urine and fæces was mortal, except in two caſes; one of which was the parotis that proved very tedious; and the other was the fortunate criſis on the eighteenth day—That patient had taken a good deal of bark in the courſe of his fever.

A ſtricture, and pain either over the eyes or at the bottoms of the orbits were dangerous. Drinking greedily, and in large draughts, were dangerous ſymptoms. A hiccup was frequently an attendant of the mortal ſymptoms, and always dangerous. A dozing with the eyes half, and the mouth wide open, were very dangerous. A deep ſighing was very dangerous. And in like manner were the pain and oppreſſion about the præcordia, and ſwelling of the hypochondria. Eruptions about the mouth were not favourable.

Upon feeling the pulſe throughout the whole fever, a diſagreeable ſenſation remained for ſome time after on the fingers—eſpecially if the ſkin was moiſt, unleſs the perſpiration was critical, and then no ſuch ſenſation was perceived.

Such were the melancholly attendants of that dreadful fever. Though, from my not having a ſufficient quantity of bark, this fever had, in a manner, its natural ſcope; yet we find in Dr. Cleghorn's very accurate account of the fever in Minorca, a few other ſymptoms of a much more malignant nature.*

An apoplexy; and though only a ſymptom of that fever, is univerſally allowed to be the moſt violent and fatal diſeaſe to which the human frame is naturally ſubject. A cholera morbus—The vomitings and purgings in the fever on board of the Weaſel were violent at times, but I think could not properly be called by that name.

A cardialgia. The pain and oppreſſion about the præcordia, or in the ſtomach, in the Weaſel's fever, did not occaſion a ſwooning away—as Blancard defines that diſeaſe or ſymptom to occaſion.

Vomiting of matter like the grounds of coffee—I did not obſerve.

A palpitation of the heart, was not complained of by any of my patients.

A pulſation of the abdominal viſcera, I never obſerved.

The pain or abſceſs in the hip never occurred to me in the Weaſel.

In theſe few circumſtances only, did the fever at Minorca and that on the coaſt of Guinea ſeem to differ, as I found upon examining that accurate writer after

* The land exhalations affected his patients; which was not the caſe on board of the Weaſel.

after I returned to England; for I was ſo unfortunate as not to have his book with me.

Reſpecting the days which were moſt critical in both forms of the fever, I muſt obſerve, that a perfect remiſſion was obtained in one caſe upon the third. A diſtinct remiſſion of thirty hours was obtained on the morning of the fifth in another caſe; but in this the fever again returned with more violence, and continued ſo twelve hours.

Four men died on the eighth; one of whom was dumb; and the parotis began to ſuppurate.

On the ninth, the critical purging began amongſt them who had the fever in its mildeſt form.

On the tenth, one died; and three on the eleventh.

The yellow ſuffuſions and purging which proved a favorable criſis to many, appeared on the thirteenth; and in one caſe an equable perſpiration broke out, which was ſucceeded the next day by a gentle diarrhæa that proved ſalutary.

One died on the fourteenth, and the parotis in another patient was ready for opening on the fifteenth.

On the ſixteenth day one died, and another was ſeized with the piles.

An unexpected criſis happened from a ſound ſleep, and a free perſpiration, on the eighteenth.

On the twenty firſt day, there was a favorable criſis of the tedious though mild fever by perſpiration.

Moſt of the ten men who died had never been in a hot climate before.

Section IV

The Method in which the Fever was treated.

I Always began with a vomit, and gave it as ſoon as the patient complained, unleſs he was then in a ſtate of perſpiration. In that caſe I encouraged the perſpiration, either with acidulated drink, or gave him ſal. nitr. and ſoon after the perſpiration was over I adminiſtered the vomit, which was the tartar emetic. —except when he had a purging, then I gave the pulv. Ipecacoan. The manner in which I adminſtered the tartar emetic, was by diſolving three grains of it in half a pint of ſimple water, of which two ſpoonfuls were taken every half hour until it began to operate, which was commonly after giving it the third or fourth time. By that means it not only vomited him well, but likewiſe often operated once, twice or oftener by ſtool; and frequently by perſpiration. Moſt commonly it was worked off with warm water.

If

If it was in the evening that they took the puke, I gave them about an hour and a half after its operation was ended, a ſaline draught with more or leſs of the eſſence of antimony, to keep up the perſpiration if there was any, or otherwiſe to promote a perſpiration; and allowed them plenty of ſage tea or barley water, either with nitre, or acidulated.*

The ſaline mixture was made after the uſual manner; ſometimes with lime juice, at other times with elixir of vitriol. I often uſed the ſpiritus Mindereri likewiſe. Thoſe mixtures were always diluted with ſimple water, ſweetened with a little ſugar, and had a due proportion of either Huxham's eſſence of antimony, or emetic tartar added to it.

But if the patient complained in the morning, ana took his vomit then, whether he had one or two ſtools therewith, I generally gave about two hours after its operation was over, an ounce of ſal. cath. amar. diſſolved in half a pint of thin water gruel, or barley water. One or other of which was ordered likewiſe for working the purge off; and if the ſkin was hot and dry towards night, I ordered the ſaline mixture before mentioned.

As the ſtomach was always loaded with bile, and the inteſtinal canal with ſaburra in the beginning of the fever, as appeared from the operation of thoſe medicines, I judged thoſe noxious contents ought quickly to be expelled, which that method effected in a gentle manner.

They who had a diarrhœa accompanying the fever, were either ordered manna with the ſalts, or rhubarb alone to purge them; and they had no ſaline mixture preſcribed, nor accid in their drink.

If it was the ſecond day before the purge was taken, the patient had no other medicine until night, when the ſaline mixture was ordered with diluting drink. Otherwiſe I uſually gave the ſaline mixture---always with one of the antimonials---every four hours, and plenty of cooling drink, with a view to procure a remiſſion. But in ſome caſes, notwithſtanding this refrigerating, relaxing, and aperient method, I was obliged to give ſmall quantities of ſalts every other day, without which they never had a ſtool, though they drank commonly tamarind beverage. In others it was neceſſary at times, to give draughts of an infuſion of camomile, to promote the diſcharge of bile upwards as nature indicated. But when the vomiting was violent or frequent, I added ſome tinct. thebaic. to the ſaline mixture, and likewiſe for the headach when it was very violent; both of which it relieved only while the effect of the doſe continued.

In this manner, the mixture with the antimonials and their drink was adminiſtered for ſeveral days, but in the caſes attended with the purging, I gave rhubarb, and ipecacoan. with opiates in ſmall doſes, and demulcent drink.

F Beſides

* I was often obliged to uſe the mineral acids for want of the vegetable acids.

Besides those, I tried at different times, when the pulse began to sink, when the headach was vehement, or other nervous symptoms appeared—the pulv. contrayerv. infus. & tinct. serp. virg. aquæ spirituosæ, sp. vol. aromat. confect. cardiac. & mosch. and I sometimes experienced the good effects of them, particularly, when blisters were likewise applied. They raised the pulse, relieved the headach, quieted the nervous spasms considerably, and removed the stupor or coma in a great measure. But bark was too often *wanted* to compleat the cure. Camphor was serviceable in one case only.

They who had the fever in its mildest form, now and then eat a little sago, thin rice gruel, or panada with a little sugar and cinnamon; but the rest would not swallow the least grain of food, until a favourable crisis was obtained.

Section V.

Cases of the remitting Fever.

CASE I.

C. P. about 32 years of age, very stout, of a healthy complexion, and had never been in a hot climate before, complained the 14th of August, *p. m.* of a sickness at the stomach, and an inclination to puke; a headach: thirst; and that he was much out of order. His pulse was very little quicker than natural, though his skin was hot and dry; and his tongue was of its natural colour. I prescribed the emetic tart. which operated very well; and at night gave him a saline draught, after the usual manner, and barley water four with nitre in it for his drink.

2d, *A. m.* He found himself rather better; but about 3 *p. m.* he turned very hot, thirsty, and uneasy. A dose of salts and manna were ordered for him; and as soon as it was worked off, the saline mixture was repeated every hours, and tamarind beverage allowed him for common drink.

3d, He spent a very bad night. His skin was very hot and dry; his countenance much flushed; the blood vessels of the tunica conjunctiva of the eyes were quite turgid; his tongue was dry and foul; and his pulse quick and full. But he complained only of being hot; that he was much out of order; and that nothing which he took had any taste. The saline mixture was well diluted, and repeated every two hours, with nitre in it, and tamarind beverage allowed for drink. He had one stool in the day.

4th, He was not quite so restless in the night, but made water several times, with a scalding; and perspired freely most part of the night. *A. m.* he was not

not quite ſo hot, and ſeemed more lively; but his tongue continued foul and though he was very thirſty, no drink pleaſed him. *P. m.* He puked ſome phlegm ſeveral times, which made him hot, and exceedingly reſtleſs, until he fell into a profuſe perſpiration each time. A violent paroyxſm followed ſoon after, with a pain and heat in his right foot; giddineſs; anxiety; and great inquietude. His pulſe was ſtrong, but not quick; his ſkin was exceeding hot, with a clammy moiſture on it, which impreſſed a very diſagreeable ſenſation on the fingers ſome time after feeling of his pulſe; and his tongue was white, dry, and chopped in the middle, with a red margin, and trembled much when he put it out. At ten *p. m.* his pulſe was extremely quick; his ſkin dry; his urine very high coloured, with a cloud at the top; he was afraid to ſleep, becauſe of frightful dreams and notions which made him ſtart out of ſhort ſlumbers; he was apprehenſive of dying; and wandered a little. He continued his mixture with the nitre (and antimonials always) in it. And at three, *p. m.* eight grains of camphor were preſcribed every three hours; and his drink was frequently changed. He had two copious ſtools.

5th, He was troubled much with inquietude in the night, and at four *a. m.* his reaching returned; after which he had a copious looſe ſtool: and perſpired freely. The fever and all the ſymptoms gradually decreaſed, and a perfect remiſſion began at noon; when his urine was ſtill high coloured, with the cloud much ſubſided, though not near to the bottom of the glaſs. This paroxyſm terminated the ſecond period of the fever. He continued his medicines, as preſcribed the preceding day, until noon; when a drachm of the pulv. cort. Peruv. was ordered every hour; but after 9, *p. m.* he only took it every two hours for the night; which agreed very well with him though only given in water, and procured him ſeveral copious ſtools.

6th, He continued cool and eaſy after a tolerable night's reſt; got up, and was ſhaved and ſhifted. He complained then of giddineſs; great weakneſs of his loins, and had no appetite. At 6 *p. m.* he found the pain and heat returning into his foot and leg; with his headach, and heat; and at 7, the fever, and all the former ſymptoms came on with increaſed violence. He took his bark regularly every two hours, until the paroxyſm commenced, when his ſtomach would not retain it. On the intermediate hours, chicken broth was allowed him, and one diſh of coffee, which he was deſirous of. Afterwards the camphor---this is the only caſe wherein the ſtomach would bear it,---the ſaline mixture, and his drink, were repeated as on the 4th.

7th, He had an exceeding bad night. *A. m.* His pulſe was ſofter; all the ſymptoms continued though he was in a ſtate of perſpiration. He raved, his head was quite light, he ſaid, and his tongue was black. At noon he fell into a very ſound ſleep, which continued till 7 *p. m.* with a moderate perſpiration. He found himſelf quite cool, and eaſy when he awoke, and never had

had another paroxyſm. His medicines were continued until he fell aſleep, and as ſoon as he awoke, a drachm of the bark was ordered every hour, which was regularly repeated throughout the night.

8th, The bark was continued afterwards, until he was perfectly recovered, and in all he took * ten ounces of it.

Before the 10th day from his being taken ill, his head was remarkably affected from the leaſt drop of wine either with his bark, or diet, which was very light. A conſiderable time after he got well, he complained of great weakneſs in his eyes; and of the pain in his foot and leg.

C A S E II.

1ſt, *M. R.* aged about 27 years, who was very healthy, though of a thin habit, and a delicate conſtitution, on the 25th of Auguſt. at noon, in feeling a boy's pulſe as he expired—of the remitting fever---received an inſtantaneous ſhock, as if he had been ſtrongly electrified, which was immediately followed by ſuch a proſtration of both his ſpirits and ſtrength, that he could with much difficulty get upon deck, or afterwards be kept from fainting for ſome time. From the commencement of the fever on board, he had taken every forenoon, a drachm of the cortex, with a little of the tincture in water, and therefore took the ſame quantity then; but though he likewiſe repeated his draught, *p. m.* his ſpirits continued greatly depreſſed; he was quite pale, towards night his memory failed him very much, he was momentarily apprehenſive of being ſurpriſed, plagued with ſilly notions, giddy at times, very little fatigued him, and he had no appetite; his pulſe was rather languid, and his ſkin hot without any perſpiration on it.

2d, His ſleep was much interrupted with frightful dreams, wandering pains, and weakneſs in his loins. *A. m.* He had no appetite, his ſkin was dry; and he had no particular complaint, though he found himſelf much indiſpoſed. However, he ſtill attended his duty, took his bark as on the 1ſt, and a glaſs of wine in the day as uſual. At night he became very hot and reſtleſs, and all his ſymptoms more violent.

3d, He was troubled with great inquietude and uneaſineſs in the night. *A. m.* in every reſpect he found himſelf worſe, when he took ſome tart. emet. which brought much bile off his ſtomach; and in two hours after, a doſe of ſalts and manna that operated very well. *P. m.* His fever, with thirſt now ſtill continued; and at bed time, he therefore took the following draught, and drank freely of weak accidulated tea through the night. Q. miſtur. ſalin. dilut.

* Doctor Lind, has omitted the three ounces which he uſed while he was in a convaleſcent ſtate; and therefore ſays, he only took ſeven ounces. See the note p. 64, of his book on hot climates.

dilut. ℥ifs. aq. cinnamom. fp. ℥i, tinct. ferp. virg. ʒii. eff. antimon. gt. xx. tinct. theb. gt. x. facch. alb. ad gratum faporem fiat hauftus.

4th, He had no fleep, though he perfpired freely, and was eafy in the night. *a. m.* his pulfe was pretty regular, his fkin cool, a fediment appeared in his urine, which was high coloured; and he was in better fpirits. He took an ounce and a half of the cortex in fix hours, and never had any return of his fever, notwithftanding he daily continued attending the fick. He did not leave off taking the cortex regularly, for a confiderable time.

SECTION VI.

Obfervations concerning the Caufe of the Fevers prevailing on board.

THE time when, and manner in which the preceding cafe occurred, puts it beyond a doubt, that remitting fevers are contagious. But I am not of opinion, that Dav. Clency, who came from the Hound Sloop, on board of the Weafel, and fell ill the day after of a true fimple Tertian---with real intermiffions, as appears from his cafe---infected the fhip's company therewith, notwithftanding the Serjeant was the very next day feized exactly with the fame fever as his; and all the Protei-form appearances---if I may be allowed the expreffion---under which remitting fevers attack: and though that excellent practitioner, Doctor Lind, upon converfing with him on that head, was inclined to think that Clency had infected our men. One would imagine from the fimilarity of the two cafes, that the Serjeant was infected from him; but he muft at that rate have caught it in the firft paroxyfm of Clency's fever; for Clency had only had one before he was feized with his. Befides, the remitting fever did not make its appearance before the Serjeant and Clency were quite well. I muft likewife add, that if it was effentially one and the fame fever---no two fevers ever differed more apparently.

What ftill confirms me more ftrongly in my opinion, is that both of his Majefty's Sloops, the Hound and Merlin, which were then at different places on the coft---the one was at Senegal, and the other at Sierra Leon---had the fame remitting fever as we had on board of the Weafel; and buried each of them the fame number of men, if I am rightly informed, without having contracted it by infection---The weather alone—or the heavy rains, &c.—in my opinion, were fufficient to occafion the fever. See the abftract thereof, pages 5th and 6th.

However, whether my reafoning on this head be fufficiently juft, or otherwife; it is by no means advanced with a defign to inculcate lefs care or caution on board of a healthy fhip, to avoid by all poffible methods, having the leaft intercourfe with fickly fhips, than is abfolutely neceffary; and much lefs to encourage them to admit a fickly perfon on board in any climate, either from a fhip, or the fhore. A very fickly man was received on board of a fhip, of which I was ſurgeon, on a remarkably healthy ſtation, out of charity, contrary to my advice, of which the conſequence proved very fatal, and the fever thereby occaſioned, continued in the ſhip for months after.

Before I conclude this part, it becomes neceſſary for me to aſſign a reaſon why I did not ſay any thing of, or even mention the bark amongſt the remedies which I made uſe of, in the general method of treatment of the fever. I know that it was the only medicine which poſſibly would have ſaved ſome of the lives of thoſe who died in it, but as I had it not to preſcribe in a ſufficient quantity to become effectual in thoſe caſes, I could not ſay, without doing much violence to my own opinion, that it failed in any of them; and therefore thought it moſt proper to omit it. Beſides, was I to advance that it failed in curing of this fever, becauſe I did give it, though not liberally enough to anſwer the purpoſe, it might be productive of much miſchief, if any younger practitioner than myſelf was thereby prevented from depending wholly, in a manner, upon the bark in curing the remittent fever hereafter.

So far from advancing any ſuch erroneous aſſertion, I thought it a duty incumbent on me to acquaint the commiſſioners for ſick and hurt, as ſoon as we arrived in England, that I was perfectly convinced moſt of the men who died of that fever had been loſt from my having too little bark; and that I had brought home ſeveral very bad caſes from the ſame cauſe, notwithſtanding I had carried out with me more than three times the quantity which was ſent on board from apothecary's hall for foreign ſervice.

But in the malignant caſes of the fever, the ſtomach would ſeldom retain a ſingle doſe without the tinct. thebaic. being joined with the cortex. However, I have ſince experienced, that with the addition of wine only, the ſtomach has been enabled to retain it when the remiſſion was very imperfect.*

I am of opinion that a reproach is frequently thrown out not only againſt the bark but other valuable remedies likewiſe, by practitioners giving them in quantities much inadequate to the diſeaſe with which they have to cope; or in a manner diſproportioned to the expectations which they form, on adminiſtering them; which are exactly the ſame in the conſequence.

If ſuch gentlemen therefore, inſtead of aſſerting poſitively in general terms, that ſuch and ſuch remedies failed in certain diſeaſes, would take the pains to relate the particulars of ſuch caſes minutely, in which they were adminiſtered, taking care to mention at the ſame time what quantity of the medicine they exhibited in a doſe, how often it was repeated, the patient's manner of living, &c. they would do more towards promoting the real knowledge of medicine than all the dogmatical aſſertions, which they could poſſibly advance, ever can; and they would be much more regarded by every gentleman of candor and eminence of the profeſſion, for ſo doing.

* See Part III

END OF THE FIRST PART.

PART II.

The Meteorological Journal, and State of the Sick Lift on board of His Majefty's Ship, Rainbow, in 1772, 1773, and 1774.

CHAPTER I.

THE DIARY OF THE WEATHER AND STATE OF THE SICK LIST, BETWEEN THE 30th OF DECEMBER 1771, AND THE 26th OF AUGUST 1772.

Year, Months, and Days.	Hours.	Thermometer	Latitude or different parts.	Longitude made.	Moon's Age.	Winds.	Rain and Dew.	Appearances of the Atmosphere.	REMARKS, AND STATE OF THE SICK LIST.
1771 Dec. 30 Die Lunæ	7 7	55 57	Off the Lizzard		24	f NE t ENE **		cl.	Sailed from Spithead yesterday about noon, in company with His Majesty's Sloop Weasel; five colds with slight fevers in the list.
31	7 7	57 57	47° 29″	From the Lizzard 03° 33″W	25	ENE ***	.	cl.	A cold added to the list; 6 in it.
1772 Jan. 1 Die Mercurii	7 12 7	57 58 57	45° 27″	06° 32″W	26	ENE ESE ***	.	cl.	Three of the colds returned to duty, and 3 remain in the list. The air is much milder.
2	7 12 7	58 61 56	42° 40″	07° 58″W	27	f ENE t SEBS ***	. .	cl.	A cold added to the list; 4 in it A cold evening.
3	7 12 7	58 57 57	39° 40″	09° 05″W	28	f ENE t SEBS ***		cl.	No alteration in the list. The colds are feverish and have a cough.
4	7 12 7	59 60 60	37° 45″	09° 48″W	29	f ENE t SEBS **		cl.	A cold added to the list; five in it. Very pleasant weather.
5	7 12 7	61 61 60	35° 22″	10° 20″W	m. a. m.	f ENE t SEBS ***	. . .	cl.	The colds—all of which proceeded from iregularities—are better. No alteration in the list.
6	7 12 7	61 64 62	33° 05″	10° 16″W	2	f ENE t SEBS ***	. . .	cl.	A cold added to the list; 6 in it. Seven p. m. we anchored at Madeira in Foncheall Bay which is very open.
7	7 12 7	63 65 63	Madeira		3	ESE **	. . .	cl.	One cold well, and another added to the list; 6 in it.
8	7 12 7	66 69 65			4	ESE **	. .	cl.	No alteration in the list.
9	7 12 7	67 71 68			5	W WBN **	. .	cl.	A contusion added to the list; 7 in it. A warm day.
10	7 12 7	68 69 68			6	f SW t NNW ***	. . .	cl.	One cold returned to duty; 6 in the list
11	7 12 7	69 70 70			7	WBN***		cl.	One of the colds is a venereal; one cold added to the list; 6 in it.

Year, Months, and Days	Hours.	Thermometer.	Latitude of different Parts.	Longitude made.	Moon's age	Winds.	Rain or Dew.	Appearances of the Atmosphere.	REMARKS, AND STATE OF THE SICK LIST.
1772 Jan. 12	7 12 7	68 71 69			8	f WbN t WSW**		c.	The contusion returned to duty; 5 in the list.
13	7 12 7	69 71 69			9	f EbN t ESE		c.	Four of the colds returned to duty: the cold remaining in the list is rheumatick.
14	7 12 7	69 71 69	Madeira		10	f EbN t ESE **		cl.	One rheumatism added to the list; 2 in it. Sailed at four p. m. in company with the Weasel.
15	7 12 7	70 71 70	30° 35″	from Madeira 00° 42″ E	11	E. ESE**		cl.	One feverish complaint added to the list; 3 in it.
16	7 12 7	70 71 69	Teneriff	00° 55″ E	12	E **		cl.	No alteration in the list. Anchor'd at 4 p. m. in St. Cruze Road, which is very open.
17	7 12 7	72 72 70			13	Nly **		c.	One feverish complaint added to the list; 4 in it, Employed watering the ship; the water very good. A. m. sultry.
18	7 12 7	73 71 69			14	Nly **	•	cl.	No alteration in the list. A. m. very sultry. A fog continually over the high land.
19	7 12 7	70 70 60			15	Nly **	•	cl.	Two feverish complaints well, and two added to the list; four in it.
20	7 12 7	70 70 69			p. a. m.	V **		c.	One contusion, and one feverish complaint added to the list; 6 in it.
21	7 12 7	70 71 71			17	V **		c.	One feverish complaint well; and one contusion added to the list; 6 in it.
22	7 12 7	72 71 70			18	f NW t WSW**		cl.	One feverish complaint well; 5 in the list. Sailed with the Weasel at 3 p. m.
23	7 12 7	72 71 70	27° 37″		19	f W t NW***		cl.	No alteration in the list.
24	7 12 7	71 71 70	24° 37″	from Teriff 00° 31 W	20	WNW**		c.	One contusion, and one rheumatism well the list.

H

Year, Months, and Days.	Hours.	Thermometer.	Latitude or different parts.	Longitude made.	Moon's age.	Winds.	Rain or Dew.	Appearances of the Atmosphere.	REMARKS, AND STATE OF THE SICK LIST.
1772 Jan. 25	7 12 7	72 71 71	22° 30″	01° 14″ W	21	f WNW t NNE **		c.	One feverifh complaint well; 2 in the lift. Very pleafant weather.
26	7 12 7	72 72 71	20° 52″	01° 12″ W	22	V **		c.	The contufion well; 1 in the lift.
27	7 12 7	72 72 72	19° 06″	00° 23″ W	23	f WNW t NE		c.	No alteration in the lift.
28	7 12 7	73 74 72	18° 05″	00° 26″ E	24	*		c.	The rheumatifm—now an ulcer—in the lift only.
29	7 12 7	74 74 73	17° 48″	00° 39″ E	25	Nly *		c.	No alteration in the lift.
30	7 12 7	74 73 73	16° 04″ Senegal	00° 22″ E	26	Nly *		c.	Only one in the lift. Anchor'd with the Weafel off Senegal Fort at noon.
31	7 12 7	74 73 72	15° 57″	From Senegal 00° 17″ W	27	N **		cl.	At 11 a. m. failed, and left the weafel. No alteraton in the lift.
Feb. 1 Die Saturni	7 12 7	73 75 73	15° 27″	03° 16″ W	28	NbE NNE **		cl.	No addition to the lift. The Thermometer was placed in the Captain's cabbin,
2	7 12 7	74 75 75	15° 11″ St. Jago	06° 04″ W	29	NNE **		c.	One in the lift. At 6 p. m. anchor'd in Praya Bay—St. Jago one of the Cape de Verde Iflands—The land round it is high except a fmall beach where boats land, beyond which is a marfhy vale where fome wells are; of which the water is very indifferent.
3	7 12 4 7	74 78 80 78	Praya Bay in 14° 52″		m. p. m.	NNE **		c.	Anchor'd rather too near a very fickly outward bound Dutch Eaft India-man; above 100 bad of the remitting fever, and dyfentery, nd buried a good many. A conftant frefh Sea breeze over the high land. The Sentinel on the booms over the water was taken ill in the night; 2 in the lift.
4	8 12 4 8	75 80 81 79			2	NNE **		c.	One feized laft night with feverifh fymptoms; 3 in the lift. Yefterday's complaint a remitting fever. P. m. very warm.
5	8 12 8	76 79 77	St. Jago			NNE **		cl.	Yefterday's complaint well, 1 contufion, and 1 fever, who was taken bad the 3d, added to the lift; 4 in it. Several of the gentlemen and men on board perceive a very difagreeable fmell from

Year, Months, and Days.	Hours.	Thermometer.	Latitude or different parts.	Longitude made.	Moon's age.	Winds.	Rain or Dew.	Appearances of the Atmosphere.	REMARKS, AND STATE OF THE SICK LIST.
1772 Feb. 5.									the Dutch Indiaman at times. Plenty of hogs, Goats, Turkies, and Fowls to be bought for old cloaths a ſhore; but they have no vegetables.
6	8 12 8	76 77 74			4	NNE **		cl.	One fever added to the liſt. Yeſterday's fever is a remittent; 5 in the liſt. 4 p. m. Sailed. The people bought a good many Hogs, Goats, &c.
7	8 12 8	74 74 74	13° 41″	from St. Jago 02° 05″ E	5	NE **		cl.	One feveriſh complaint added to the liſt; 6 in it.
8	8 12 8	74 73 73	11° 49″	04° 49″ E	6	NE **		cl.	Two feveriſh complaints added to the liſt; 8 in it. The feveriſh complaints are ſlight remittents.
9	8 12 8	73 72 74	10° 06″	07° 07″ E	7	NE *	❖	cl.	One feveriſh complaint added, the 6th and the one of the 7th well, 1 with eruptions added to liſt; 7 in it.
10	8 12 8	72 72 75	09° 09″	08° 26″ E	8	NE *	❖	cl.	One ſlight indiſpoſition added to the liſt; 8 in it.
11	8 12 8	75 78 77	08° 44″	09° 36″ E	9	NE *	❖	cl.	The contuſion and 1 with eruptions well; and 1 feveriſh complaint added to the liſt; 7 in it. At 9 p. m. anchor'd off Sierra Leon River.
12	8 12 8	78 79 80	Cape Sierra Leon. 08° 30″		10	NE *	❖	h.	At 6 a. m. failed, and anchored at 5 p. m. in Sierra Leon river. The indiſpoſition of the 10th well, and 1 lame added to the liſt; 7 in it.
13	8 12 4 8	78 80 81 80			11	Sb & lb	❖	h.	One added to the liſt with feveriſh complaints; 8 in it. The Sea breeze blows over part of the land which is covered with thick trees and ſhrubs, with a fogg always over them; which becomes thick towards ſun ſet. The land breeze blows from high hills covered in the ſame manner, which can ſeldom be ſeen for fog.
14	8 12 4 8	80 81 82 80			12	Sb & lb	❖	h.	Two fevers well, 1 of them bad remittents; 6 in the liſt Our watering tent fixed aſhore on the beach which is overflown at high water; and emits noxious exhalations when the tide leaves it. A gentleman and eight men ſleep in the tent; and in the night it is covered with fog. It is always hazy on the river though the ſun ſhines.
15	8 12 4 8	80 81 82 80			13	Sb & lb	❖	h.	The feveriſh complaint of the 13th well, 5 in the liſt. A party of the men go aſhore every day to cut wood; but come on board at night. Very good water here, unleſs in the rainy ſeaſons, when it is thick.

Year, Months, and Days.	Hours.	Thermometer.	Latitude or different parts.	Longitude made.	Moon's Age.	Winds.	Rain and Dew.	Appearances of the Atmosphere.	REMARKS, AND STATE OF THE SICK LIST.
1772 Feb. 16	8 12 4 8	79 80 81 79			14	Sb & lb	✣	h.	The lame complaint well; 4 in the list. Plenty of fish in the river, but no stock, and very few vegetables to be got ashore; which is chiefly owing to the indolence of the natives.
17	8 12 8	79 80 80			15	Sb & lb	✣	h.	One feverish complaint returned to duty; 3 in the list. Very heavy dews.
18	8 12 4 8	78 79 81 79			p. p. m.	Sb & lb *	✣	h.	No alteration in the list.
19	8 12 4 8	79 79 81 79			17	Sb & lb	✣	h.	One feverish complaint, 2 diarrhœa, 1 with eruptions, and 1 cough added to the list; 1 of the remitting fevers and 1 of the feverish complaints well; 6 in the list.
20	8 12 4 8	79 79 81 79			18	Sb & lb	✣	h.	Yesterday's feverish complaint well; and 3 added to the list; 8 in it.
21	8 12 8	79 80 80			19	Sb & lb	✣	h.	One of the diarrhœa of the 19th well; 7 in the list.—The Sea and land breezes are very irregular.
22	8 12 8	80 79 80	Sierra Leon		20	Sb & lb	✣	cl. h.	A deaf complaint added to the list; 8 in it.
23	8 12 8	78 79 79			21	Sb & lb	✣	h. cl.	A feverish complaint of the 19th well. The Weasel came in. Her men were seized with catarrhous complaints while they lay at Senegal from thick foggy, disagreeable weather, and are not yet well.
24	8 12 8	79 80 80			22	Sb & lb	✣	h. cl.	Seven in the list. The dews are less than they were.
25	8 12 8	79 81 80			23	Sb & lb	✣	h. cl.	One diarrhœa of the 19th, and 1 feverish of the 20th well; 5 in the list. None of the Weasel's men sleep ashore.
26	8 12 8	80 81 81			24	Sb & lb	✣	h. cl.	A fever of the 20th well; 4 in the list. Every person on board complains of their sleep not refreshing them.
27	8 12 8	80 80 80	08° 13″		25	f WNW t NWbW	✣	h. cl.	One fever of the 20th, and one with eruptions well; p. m. a slight complaint well. 1 griped, and 1 feverish complaint added. 3 bad.

Year, Months, and Days.	Hours.	Thermometer	Latitude or different parts.	Longitude made.	Moon's Age.	Winds.	Rain and Dew.	Appearances of the Atmosphere.	REMARKS, AND STATE OF THE SICK LIST.
1772 Feb. 28	8 12 8	80 80 80	07° 10″	from Sierra Leon 00° 23″W	26	N NNE *		h. cl.	One feverifh complaint added to the lift; 4 in it. A few flight fun-burned complaints not in the lift.
29	8 12 8	80 80 80	06° 40″	00° 48″ E	27	V p. m. ⁂	. .	h. cl.	Two fevers added to the lift—one of them came on board from a merchantman at Sierra Leon—6 in it. 3 Fevers; 1 griped, 1 ulcer, and 1 deaf complaint.
Martii 1 Die Sabbati	8 12 8	79 80 79	06° 26″	01° 58″ E	28	f NNE t NNW **	❖	h. cl.	The feverifh complaint added the 27th ult. is a bad remittent—he was one of the watering party at Sierra Leon, 2 feverifh, and 2 griped complaints added to the lift; 10 in it.
2	8 12 8	79 80 80	05° 40″	02° 40″ E	29	f WNW t N *	❖	h. cl.	One of yefterday's feverifh complaints came from a merchant-man at Sierra Leon—he and the other man were exceedingly nafty when they came on board, and they complained of being ftarved on board of the fhip which they came from; the 1 added to the lift the 29th ult. is a bad remitting fever; 10 in the lift.
3	8 12 8	81 79 81	05° 20″ Going along fhore		30	f NNW t ESE *	❖	h. cl.	Two flight complaints well, and 1 added to the lift. The feverifh complaint added the 1ft from the merchant-man is an eryfipelas; 9 in the lift. 4 of them are bad remittents; 3 of which were of the watering party at Sierra Leon. Always hazy though the fun fhines.
4	8 12 4 8	79 80 83 81	04° 46″		m. a. m.	f NWbW t NE	❖	h. cl.	Another waterer added to the lift with a fever; 10 in it. Every thing very damp and mouldy on board; and wood fhrinks amazingly. The fails mildewed very much.
5	8 12 8	80 80 82	04° 20″		2	V *	❖	h. cl.	No alteration in the lift. The Weafel's men have had bilious gripings fince we left Sierra Leon. It cannot be from the water becaufe our men have the fame. Very heavy dews.
6	8 12 8	80 82 80	04° 15″		3	V *	❖	h. cl.	A waterer added to the lift with a fever; and a feverifh complaint laft night. P. m. The old ulcer and one flight fever well, 2 feverifh complaints added to the lift; 12 in it.
7	8 12 8	80 80 81	04° 16″		4	V *	❖	h. cl.	One waterer, a fever—1 feverifh, one of the wooders, and 1 griped complaints, added to the lift; 15 in it— 2 of them flight.
8	8 12 8	80 80 78	04° 36″		5	V *	❖	h. cl.	No alteration in the lift. The evening very cool.
9	8 12 8	78 78 79	04° 54″ along fhore		6	V **	❖	h. cl.	Two flight complaints, the eryfipelas, and the lame complaint well; 11 in the lift 7 of them very bad remittents, fix of whom were of the watering party. The wind moftly off the land, which is very uncommon here. The day cold.

Year, Months, and Days.	Hours.	Thermometer.	Latitude or different Parts.	Longitude made.	Moon's age.	Winds.	Rain or Dew.	Appearances of the Atmosphere.	REMARKS, AND STATE OF THE SICK LIST.
1772 Martii 10	8 12 8	79 80 81	05° 02″	from Cape Lehou 00° 32″ E	7	V *	❖	h. cl.	One headach and naufea, an old complaint—added to the lift. P. m. The wooder, and the griped complaints of the 7th well; 10 bad.
11	8 12 8	81 81 82	05° 05″	01° 42″ E	8	V *	❖	h. cl.	One griped complaint added to the lift; 11 in it.
12	8 12 4 8	82 82 83 82	04° 57″ Appalonia		9	SSW **	❖	h.	Two diarrhœa, and 1 of the waterers with a fever added to the lift; 14 in it. Some flight feverifh complaints not in the lift. From 1 to 3 p. m. we were anchored off Appalonia, where we left the Weafel. A hot day.
13	8 12 4 8	82 82 83 82	05° 00″ Dick's Cove		10	SW *	❖	h. cl.	One of yefterday's diarrhœa well; 13 in the lift. A. m. we anchored off Dick's Cove, and failed at 5 p. m.
14	8 12 4 8	82 83 84 87	Cape Coaft.		11	a. m. V *		h. cl.	The other diarrhœa of the 12th well. At noon anchored at Cape Coaft. 5 P. m. I carried the Thermometer down into my cabbin in the Cock Pit.
15	8 12 8	87 82 81			12	Sb & lb **		h. c.	One guinea worm, and one abfcefs added to the lift; 14 in it. 9 A. m. brought up the thermometer to the Captain's cabbin again. The Sea breeze blows frefh; but there is very little wind in the night. Though feemingly a paradox, it is true, that it is hazy though the fun fhines bright, and no clouds.
16	8 12 8	81 81 80			13	Sb & lb **		h. c.	No alteration in the lift. The thermometer in the caftle—in the fhade—is generally at this time of the year between 82 and 85, and higheft at noon I am informed.
17	8 12 8	82 84 83			14	Sb & lb **	. .	h. cl.	One feverifh of the 7th; 1 of the 12th; and a diarrhœa with gripes, well; 1 diarrhœa with a naufea, and 1 feverifh complaint added to the lift; 13 in it. The Weafel came in.
18	8 12 8	79 8 79			15	V *	. .	cl.	One added to the lift with the piles; 14 in it. As foon as the Tornado began the thermometer fell.
19	8 12 4 8	78 8 83 82			p. a. m.	V **		cl.	No alteration in the lift. The only vegetables to be bought is yams, and they are not plenty. Limes are very fcarce.
20	8 12 4 8	81 81 84 83			17	V **		cl.	The headach of the 10th well; 1 furuncle, and 1 lame complaint added to the lift; 15 in it. P. m. very hot.

Year, Months, and Days.	Hours.	Thermometer.	Latitude or different parts.	Longitude made.	Moon's age.	Winds.	Rain or Dew.	Appearances of the Atmosphere.	REMARKS, AND STATE OF THE SICK LIST.
1772 Martii 21	8 12 8	83 83 81			18	V **		cl.	The abfcefs of the 15th, the feverifh of the 17th, and yefterday's complaints well, 1 naufea with a cough added to the lift; 13 in it.
22	8 12 4 8	81 82 83 81			19	V **		cl.	A fever of the 6th well; 12 in the lift. It is only cloudy at times.
23	8 12 4 8	79 82 87 f. 84			20	V **		cl.	The feverifh returned 21ft, relapfed; 13 in th lift.
24	8 12 8	83 84 84			21	V **		cl. l.	No alteration in the lift.
25	8 12 8	82 84 84			22	V **		c.	The naufea of the 21ft well; 12 in the lift—A very few fowls only to be got here at prefent—and no other ftock.
26	8 12 8	81 82 82	p. m. Anamaboe		23	V *		cl.	The relapfed of the 23d well; 11 in the lift. Sailed at 5 p. m. and at 8 p. m. anchor'd at Anamaboe.
27	8 12 8	82 84 83	Tantum Querrie		24	V *		cl.	The fever of the 3d, and the piles of the 18th, well; 9 in the lift. Sailing down the coaft, and touching at the Forts.
28	8 12 5 8	83 84 85 83	Winnebah		25	S **		cl.	The darrhœa of the 17th, and the furuncle of the 20th well; 2 headachs added to the lift; 9 in it.
29	8 12 4 8	82 82 83 83	Accra		26	V **		cl. h.	The 2 fevers of the 29th ult. the fever of the 4th, and the fever of the 6th, well; 5 in the lift.
30	8 12 4 8	79 83 84 82			27	W **		h. cl.	No alteration in the lift. The people were healthy at every place we called at, it being their healthy feafon; but fome have habitual tertians which they feemed to pay little regard to.
31	8 12 4 8	80 81 83 82			28	V **		h. cl.	One headach of the 28th well, and 1 added to the lift; 5 in it. 1 Tertian recovering, 2 headachs, 1 guinea worm, and 1 lame. At noon took our departure from the coaft, with the Weafel.
Aprilis 1 Die Mercurii	8 12 8	82 84 83	04° 1	from Accra 01° 06″ E.	29	f SSW t WSW **		h. cl.	The lame complaint does duty, and a headach added to the lift; 5 in it.

Year, Months, and Days.	Hours.	Thermometer.	Latitude or different parts.	Longitude made.	Moon's age.	Winds.	Rain or Dew.	Appearances of the Atmosphere.	REMARKS, AND STATE OF THE SICK LIST.
1772 Aprilis 2	8 12 8	83 83 84	03° 17″	01° 56″ E	30	f SWbS t SbW *		h. cl.	Two headachs well; 1 griped complaint, 1 cold, suppressed perspiration—and 1 contusion added to the list; 6 in it.
3	8 12 4 8	83 83 85 84	02° 45″	02° 22″ E	m. a. m.	f SWbS t SbW **		cl.	The headach well; and 1 feverish complaint added to the list; 6 in it.
4	8 12 4 8	83 83 85 83	02° 17″	03° 20″ E	2	f SWbS t SbW *		cl.	The cold well; 1 cough, and 1 headach added to the list; 7 in it. Very hot and cloudy at times only.
5	8 12 8	84 83 83	01° 59″	04° 03″ E	3	W *		c.	Yesterday's headach; and the feverish of the 3d, well; 5 in the list.
6	8 12 8	83 82 79	01° 20″	04° 57″ E	4	V ⁂	. . .	cl. p.m.	No alteration in the list. The men all got wet.
7	8 12 8	81 83 82	00° 59″	04° 28″ E	5	S *		h.	The griped complaint of the 2d, well; 4 in the list.
8	8 12 8	82 82 83	00° 07″	05° 22″ E	6	V *		h.	Two headachs and 1 contusion added to the list; 7 in it.
9	8 12 4 8	81 81 82 81	00° 17″	06° 32″ E	7	W		h.	One cold, a suppressed perspiration, added to the list; 8 in it.
10	8 12 4 8	82 82 83 82	00° 22″	06° 51″ E	8	W *		l. h.	No alteration in the list. Anchor'd at St. Thomas's 5 p. m. together with the Weasel.
11	8 12 4 8	81 82 83 82	St. Thomas's island.		9	Sb & lb *	. .	h.	The contusion of the 8th well; 7 in the list. The town is built on the leewardmost part of the island which is not at all cleared of the woods; nor the marshes drained; the consequence of which is, it is generally peopled from Portugal every 2d year, it proves so fatal to Europeans. They are very sickly now. The water very good unless in the rainy season when it is quite thick.
12	8 12 4 8	82 82 84 03			10	Sb & lb *		h.	No alteration in the list. Plenty of Goats, Hogs, Turkies, and Fowls, to be bought a shore for old cloaths; they have likewise Yams, Bananas, and Limes, to sell in the same manner.

Year, Months, and Days.	Hours.	Thermometer.	Latitude or different Parts.	Longitude made.	Moon's age.	Winds.	Rain or Dew.	Appearances of the Atmoſphere.	REMARKS, AND STATE OF THE SICK LIST.
1772 Aprilis 13	8 12 4 8	81 82 84 83			11	Sb & lb		h.	Our men employed in wooding and watering the ſhip, but all ſleep on board. No alteration in the liſt. The iſland abounds in Guinea ſparrows.
14	8 12 8	83 84 81	St. Thomas's iſland.		12	※ p. m	. . . .	cl.	One of the headachs of the 8th well; and 1 lame complaint added to the liſt; 7 in it. The Tornado roſe ſuch a ſwell that a boat could not land on the beach to bring the men on board at night. But the gentleman who commanded the watering party at Sierra Leon—being aſhore taking a walk—ſwam off to the boat, ſo much he dreaded the conſequence of lying aſhore again.
15	8 12 8	80 79 81			13	W *	a. m.	cl.	Three complained with headachs, and a ſickneſs at ſtomach; 10 in the liſt. Above 50 of the men lay aſhore laſt night in an exceedingly damp houſe, which lies very low with a large ſwamp, the oozy beach, and a river over hung with trees and ſhrubs, cloſe to it; and are all ſurrounded with very thick woods, and ſhrubs, that are conſtantly damp, and covered with a thick fog in the night. They made large fires in the houſe and ſmoaked. Both officers and men thought ſome tincture of bark which I ſent them aſhore this morning—the captain ſent them wine to take it in—of very great benefit to them.—A number of the Weaſel's men were aſhore too.
16	8 12 4 8	80 83 84 82			14	N p. m. *		cl.	The contuſion of the 2d, the other headach of the 8th, and the cold of the 11th well; 1 contuſion added to the liſt; 8 in it.
17	8 12 4 8	82 84 86 83			p. p. m.	Sb & lb *		cl.	Three of the men who lay aſhore complained, with bilious vomitings, and a purging—2 of the headachs of the 15th well, 9 in the liſt. P. m. very hot.
18	8 12 4 8	82 83 85 82			16	SE *	. .	cl.	One of yeſterday's complaints well; 2 ſlight fevers, and 1 diarrhœa added to the liſt; 11 in it. The men buy a good many fowls, &c.
19	8 12 4 8	83 83 79 81			17	※ m.	. . .	c.	One headach with vomiting added to the liſt; 12 in it. 1 of them is a ſlight complaint. Some of the men were aſhore during the Tornado, and got wet. Got 2 bullocks on board for the ſhip's company.
20	8 12 4 8	81 83 84 83			18	Sb & lb *		cl.	The oldeſt Sierra Leon remittent, the headach of the 15th, and the contuſion of the 16th, well, 9 in the liſt.

Year, Months, and Days.	Hours.	Thermometer	Latitude or different parts.	Longitude made.	Moon's age.	Winds.	Rain or Dew.	Appearances of the Atmoſphere.	REMARKS, AND STATE OF THE SICK LIST.
1772 Aprilis 21	8 12 4 8	82 81 77 80			19	a. m. ✳	. . .	cl.	One of the complaints of the 17th; and the ſlight complaint well. 1 of the gentlemen who lay aſhore, was ſeized laſt night with a bilious vomiting, and purging; 8 in the liſt. Sailed in company with the Weaſel at 4 p. m.
22	8 12 8	82 83 82	00° 30″		20	V *		h.	One of the ſlight fevers, and the diarrhœa of the 18th, and yeſterday's complaint, well; 5 in the liſt.
23	8 12 8	81 79 79	00° 05″		21	a. m. ✳ p. m. V	. . . .	cl.	The other ſlight fever of the 18th well. 1 who went a fiſhing at St. Thomas's complained of a headach—with feveriſh ſymptoms—5 in the liſt. The Tornados always blow from the S.E.
24	8 12 8	81 83 82	00° 04″ N	from St. Thomas's 01° 20″ W	22	V *		cl.	One of the complaints of the 17th, the headach of the 19th, and yeſterday's complaint well; 1 lame complaint from a guinea worm, added to the liſt; 3 in it.
25	8 12 4 8	82 84 85 f. 84	00° 09″ S	00° 58″ W	23	V *		cl.	Two who lay aſhore added to the liſt with fevers; 5 in it.
26	8 12 8	83 83 82	00° 14″ S	01° 27″ W	24	V *	.	cl.	Two nauſeæ, and 1 aſthmatick complaint with an intermittent fever—from the Weaſel—added to the liſt; 8 in it.
27	8 12 8	82 82 82	00° 41″	02° 10″ W	25	S *		cl.	Two who lay aſhore added to the liſt with fevers, and the lame complaint of the 14th well; 9 in the liſt. Thoſe added on the 25th are very bad remittents.
28	8 12 8	82 82 81	01° 12″	03° 35″ W	26	S *		cl.	One boy who lay aſhore added to the liſt with a fever; 10 in the liſt.
29	8 12 8	81 82 82	01° 45″	04° 48″ W	27	V *		cl.	Two who lay aſhore added with fevers—all the ſhorers that are in the liſt are bad remittents—and 2 other ſlight fevers added to the liſt; 14 in it.
30	8 12 8	82 82 81	02° 10″	05° 52″ W	28	V *	a. m.	cl.	One who lay aſhore, a fever, and 1 with feveriſh complaints, added to the liſt; 16 in it. The ſhorers added yeſterday, and one of the other complaints are remitting fevers.
Maii 1 Die Veneris	8 12 8	81 82 82	03° 12″	06° 50″ W	29	V **	. .	cl.	The 2 nauſeæ of the 26th ult. and the other complaint of the 29th, well; three who lay aſhore, and 1 other complaint, added to the liſt with fevers; 17 in the liſt. 10 bad remitting fevers, 4 ſlight fevers, 1 aſthma or ague, 1 guinea worm, and 1 ulcer. Parted company with the Weaſel, 10 of her men who lay aſhore at St. Thomas's, bad.
2	8 12 8	81 81 81	03° 45″	09° 15″ W	m. p. m.	V *	. .	cl.	One added with feveriſh complaints to the liſt; 18 in it. 3 of yeſterday's complaints bad tertians, and to day's, was one of the boat's crew who had been very often wet at St. Thomas's. Cloudy at times only.

Year, Months, and Days.	Hours.	Thermometer.	Latitude or different parts.	Longitude made.	Moon's age.	Winds.	Rain or Dew.	Appearances of the Atmosphere.	REMARKS, AND STATE OF THE SICK LIST.
1772 Maii 3	8 12 8	81 80 81	03° 48″	11° 36″W	1	V *	..	cl.	The complaint of the 1ſt, who was not a ſhorer well; 17 in the liſt. Yeſterday's complaint is a remitting fever.
4	8 12 8	81 81 80	04° 05″ R.	13° 57″ W	2	SE **	.	cl.	The one added with feveriſh complaints the 30th, well; and 1 added to the liſt with piles; 17 in it.
5	8 12 8	81 82 f. 82	04° 20″	16° 43″ W	3	SE **	.	cl.	The remittent of the 29th, who was not one of the ſhorers, died a. m. unexpectedly. He was expoſed a good deal to the ſun in boats at St. Thomas's. There never was a remiſſion of his fever: 1 ſlight complaint added to the liſt; 17 in it.
6	8 12 8	80 80 80	04° 20″	19° 37″W	4	ESE **		cl.	One of the ſhorers of the 25th ult. well; 16 in the liſt. Cloudy at times only.
7	8 12 8	82 80 80	04° 20″	22° 06″ W	5	ESE *		cl.	The Weaſel's intermittent, a very old complaint who came on board of us purpoſely to be longer in a hot climate for his recovery—1 ſhorer of the 27th ult. 1 of the 1ſt, and the 1 of the 2d, all returned to duty; 12 in the liſt.
8	8 12 8	82 80 80	04° 25″	23° 43″ W	6	V *		c.	One ſhorer with feveriſh ſymptoms, and 1 headach, added to the liſt. The other ſhorer of the 25th, and 1 of the 27th ult. well; 12 in the liſt.
9	8 12 8	80 80 80	04° 11″	25° 47″ W	7	SE **		c.	The laſt piles caſe is a pox; 11 in the liſt.
10	8 12 8	81 81 81	03° 18″	27° 13″ W	8	SE. E **		cl.	The complaint of the 28th, the ſhorer of the 30th ult. and the headach of the 8th well; 1 ſhorer added to the liſt with feveriſh ſymptoms; 9 in the liſt. The ſhorer of the 8th a ſlight remittent.
11	8 12 8	81 81 81	01° 55″	29° 04″W	9	SE **		cl.	One of the ſhorers of the 29th, and the cough of the 4th ult. well; 7 in the liſt. Spoke a Portugueſe ſhip.
12	8 12 8	81 80 81	00° 36″ S	30° 00″ W	10	V **		cl.	The ſhorer of the 8th well; 6 in the liſt. Cloudy at times.
13	8 12 8	81 81 81	01° 50″ N.	from St Thomas's 30° 19″W	11	SEbS *	.	cl.	One of the ſhorers of the 29th ult. well; 5 in the liſt.
14	8 12 8	81 80 80	02° 25″	30° 38″W	12	a. m. — p. m. N	p. m. ..	cl.	The ſhorer of the 10th well; a coxſwain who was often wet in the boat at St. Thomas's added to the liſt with feveriſh ſymptoms; 5 in it.

Year, Months, and Days.	Hours.	Thermometer	Latitude or different parts.	Longitude made.	Moon's Age	Winds.	Rain and Dew.	Appearances of the Atmosphere.	REMARKS, AND STATE OF THE SICK LIST.
1772 Maii 15	8 12 8	81 81 81	04° 08″	31° 58″ W	13	V *		cl c.	Two of the shorers of the 1st, and yesterday's complaint, well; 1 nausea added to the list; 5 in it. Cloudy at times.
16	8 12 8	81 81 81	04° 44″	33° 58″ W	14	NE **	. .	cl. c.	Yesterday's complaint well; 2 in the list.
17	8 12 8	81 81 81	06° 01″	35° 50″ W	p. a. m.	V *	. .	cl. c.	Two of the shorers who were well got intermittents, 1 cough, and 1 with feverish symptoms added to the list; 6 in it.
18	8 12 8	81 80 80	07° 12″	38° 08″ W	16	NE **	❖	cl. c.	No alteration in the list. Heavy dews.
19	8 12 8	80 80 80	08° 38″	40° 22″ W	17	NE **	❖	cl. c.	The feverish complaint of the 17th an intermittent; 6 in the list. Cloudy at times.
20	8 12 8	79 79 80	10° 01″	42° 46″ W	18	NE **	❖	cl. c.	The Weasel's man relapsed, and 1 cough added to the list; 8 in it.
21	8 12 8	79 80 79	11° 19″	45° 06″ W	19	NE **	❖	c. cl.	No alteration in the list.
22	8 12 8	78 78 78	12° 08″	47° 00″ W	20	NE **	❖	c. cl.	Eight in the list. Very cold air.
23	8 12 8	78 78 78	12° 59″	48° 59″ W	21	NE **	❖	c. cl.	The cough of the 20th well; and 1 of the shorers who recovered of his remittent, seized with an intermittent fever; 8 in the list.
24	8 12 8	79 80 79	13° 05″	50° 51″ W	22	V **	❖	c. cl.	No alteration in the list. Very little dew.
25	8 12 8	81 80 79	13° 17″	52° 45″ W	23	Ely **	❖	c. cl.	The ulcer of the 24th ult. does duty; 7 in the list.
26	8 12 8	81 80 80	13° 17″	55° 08″ W	24	E	❖	c. cl.	No alteration in the list. The air now agreeably hot.
27	8 12 8	80 81 81	15° 07″	57° 45″ W	25	E NWbW **		c. cl.	The intermittents recover slowly.

Year, Months, and Days.	Hours.	Thermometer.	Latitude or different Parts.	Longitude made.	Moon's age.	Winds.	Rain or Dew.	Appearances of the Atmosphere.	REMARKS, AND STATE OF THE SICK LIST.
1772 Maii 28	8 12 8	81 81 81	16° 26″	60° 29″W	26	ENE S ***		c. cl.	Seven in the lift.
29	8 12 8	81 81 81	16° 46″ p. m. Antigua		27	V **		c. cl.	No alteration in the lift yet. At 6 p. m. anchor'd in Englifh harbour Antigua; it is very fmall and furrounded with high hills which keep the Sea breeze off, and render it very unhealthy.
30	8 12 8	80 81 81			28	ENE *		c. cl.	Seven in the lift. Admiral Mann commands here, five of His Majefty's fhips in the harbour.
31	8 12 8	81 83 82			29	SE *		c.	Sent 1 pox, and 1 very foul ulcer who came from a guineaman to the hofpital. The Weafel's man returned to duty; 6 in the lift.
Junii 1 Die Lunæ	8 12 4 8	82 83 84 83			m. a m.	SE *		c.	One of the men was killed p. m. by a fall from the main top maft head upon the quarter deck. He breathed only a few times on the deck. No wound appeared about his head; but his left leg was broke in two parts, of which 1 of the fractures was compound. The men drink new rum immoderately; 6 in the lift. 4 Intermittents, 1 guinea worm; and 1 cough.
2	8 12 8	82 82 83			2	SE *		c.	A feverifh complaint added to the lift; 7 in it. The thermometer afhore at the hofpital was 87 at 2 p. m.
3	8 12 8	82 82 80			3	SE *		c.	Two of the intermittents well; 1 with feverifh fymptoms, and 1 contufion, added to the lift; 7 in it. Sailed at 4 p. m.
4	8 12 8	80 82 82	St. Chriftopher		4	EbS **		c.	One of the intermittents well; and 1 contufion added to the lift. At 9 a. m. anchored in Baffa Terre road, and p. m. dropped down to Old road.
5	8 12 8	82 83 82			5	E **		c.	Two lame, and 1 feverifh complaints added to the lift; 10 in it. Employed watering the fhip. The water is very good.
6	8 12 8	81 83 82	17° 17″		6	E **	a. m. . . .	c. cl.	The guineaworm, and the intermittent, well. The intermittent returned to duty the 4th, has a headach from wafhing; 2 from drinking added to the lift with feverifh fymptoms; 1 of them was St. Thomas's remittent, and 1 contufion. 12 in the lift. Sailed at 6 a. m.
7	8 12 8	83 81 81	17° 18″	From St. Chriftophers 02° 28″W	7	EbN *		cl.	The 1 added with feverifh fymptoms the 3d, well; 11 in the lift.
8	8 12 8	83 81 81	17° 22″	04° 27″W	8	EbN E *	.	c. cl.	The complaint of the 2d, and the 2 feverifh ones of the 6th, well. 8 in the lift.

Year, Months, and Days.	Hours.	Thermometer.	Latitude or different parts.	Longitude made.	Moon's age.	Winds.	Rain or Dew.	Appearances of the Atmosphere.	REMARKS, AND STATE OF THE SICK LIST.
1772 Junii 9	8 12 8	85 83 82	17° 32″	06° 57″W	9	EbS **	. . .	cl.	One contusion added to the list; 9 in it. The Thermometer's being highest in the morning is owing to the sun shining in at the cabbin windows, though not upon it.
10	8 12 8	82 83 82	17° 24″	08° 48″ W	10	f SE t NE *	. . .	cl.	The contusion of the 6th, well; the Weasel's man relapsed again, and 1 with feverish symptoms added to the list; 10 in it.
11	8 12 8	83 83 82	17° 59″ Hispainiola		11	E *		c.	Two lame complaints added; the 5th well; 8 in the list. The feverish complaint added yesterday is a remitting fever, he was ailing once before, and was one of the shorers at St. Thomas's.
12	8 12 8	84 83 82	18° 14″		12	f EbS t SEbE		c.	The feverish complaint added to the list the 5th, well; 7 in the list.
13	8 12 8	83 82 82	P. m. Port Royal Jamaica.		13	V		c.	The intermittent relapsed who was returned to duty the 6th, and 3 diarrhœæ added to the list; the contusion of the 9th well; 10 in the list. At 3 p. m. anchored. Sir George Rodney commands here; 4 sail of the line, besides frigates and sloops.
14	8 12 8	83 85 82			14	Sb & lb		c.	The tertian added to the list the 10th, well; and an ulcer added to the list; 10 in it. The ships are allowed fresh meat once a week.
15	8 12 8	83 84 83			a. m. p.	Sb & lb			Sent the 2 intermittents, the Weasel's man, (and 1 ulcer and a gout, neither of whom was in the list) to the hospital; 7 in the list. The men drink immoderately of new rum.
16	8 12 8	83 84 83			16	Sb & lb		c.	The contusion of the 3d, and one of the diarrhœæ of the 13th, well; and a rheumatism added to the list; 6 in it. The Sea breeze blows so regularly here in the day, that it is called the Doctor from its being so refreshing; but the land breeze is unhealthy. The situation of Port Royal for receiving the whole benefit of the former, and being well out of the reach of the latter, renders it remarkably healthy.
17	8 12 8	83 84 83			17	Sb & lb	p. m. . . .	c. cl.	The contusion of the 3d, and 1 of the diarrhœæ of the 13th, well; 1 lumbago added to the list; 5 in it.
18	8 12 8	83 85 85			18	Sb & lb		c.	No alteration in the list.
19	8 12 4 8	82 85 86 84			19	Sb & lb		c.	One complaint with gripes added to the list; 6 in it.

Year, Months, and Days.	Hours.	Thermometer.	Latitude or different parts.	Longitude made.	Moon's age.	Winds.	Rain or Dew.	Appearances of the Atmosphere.	REMARKS, AND STATE OF THE SICK LIST.
1772 Junii 20	8 12 4 8	83 85 86 85			20	Sb & lb		c.	The rheumatism, an eryfipelas, fent to the hofpital, 1 contufion, and 1 with feverifh fymptoms added to the lift; 7 in it.
21	8 12 8	83 85 85			21	Sb & lb		c.	One contufion, and 1 drunken complaint added to the lift; 9 in it.
22	8 12 8	84 86 85			22	Sb & lb		c.	The lumbago of the 17th, the contufion of the 20th, and yefterday's complaint from drunkennefs, well; 1 with feverifh fymptoms added to the lift, 7 in it.
23	8 12 4 8	83 86 87 85			23	Sb & lb	.	c. cl.	The feverifh complaint of the 20th, the contufion of the 21ft, and a flight complaint, well; 4 in the lift. A very hot day.
24	8 12 8	84 86 85			24	Sb & lb		c. cl.	One with feverifh fymptoms added to the lift; 5 in it.
25	8 12 4 8	83 85 86 84			25	Sb & lb		c. cl.	One diarrhœa added to the lift; 6 in it.
26	8 12 8	82 85 84			26	Sb & lb		c. cl.	The feverifh complaint of the 22d, well; 5 in the lift.
27	8 12 4 8	82 84 85 84			27	Sb & lb		c. cl.	The old cough of the 4th April, and the other diarrhœa of the 13th, well; 1 contufion, and 1 cold fuppreffed perfpiration from fleeping on deck, added to the lift; 5 in it.
28	8 12 8	82 85 84			28	Sb & lb		cl. c.	The griped complaint of the 19th, and the purging of the 25th well; 1 headach, and 1 inflamation added to the lift; 5 in it.
29	8 12 8	80 85 84			29	Sb & lb		cl. c.	The feverifh complaint of the 24th, and the cold of the 27th, well; 3 in the lift.
30	8 12 8	82 84 83			m. p. m	Sb & lb		c. cl.	One diarrhœa, the feverifh complaint returned yefterday to duty, and 1 wound added to the lift; 5 in it. 1 headach, 1 inflammation, 1 wound, 1 contufion, and 1 griped complaint.
Julii 1 Die Mercurii	8 12 8	82 85 83			1	Sb & lb		c. cl.	One with feverifh fymptoms, and an inflamed leg added to the lift; 7 in it.

Year, Months, and Days.	Hours.	Thermometer	Latitude or different parts.	Longitude made.	Moon's Age	Winds.	Rain and Dew.	Appearances of the Atmosphere.	REMARKS, AND STATE OF THE SICK LIST.
1772 Julii 2	8 12 4 8	83 85 86 84			2	Sb & lb		c.	The diarrhœa, and the wound of the 30th ult. well; 1 contusion added to the list; 6 in it.
3	8 12 8	83 85 82			3	Sb & lb		c.	The contusion of the 27th, the inflammation of the 28th, and the feverish complaint of the 1st, well; 3 in the list.
4	8 12 8	82 84 82			4	Sb & lb		c.	All the seven complaints sent to the hospital, come on board, 5 of them added to the sick list; 8 in it.
5	8 12 8	82 84 83			5	Sb & lb		c.	No alteration in the list.
6	8 12 8	82 83 82	17° 36″		6	ESE **		c.	Two with feverish symptoms added to the list; 10 in it, besides a number of ulcers. 5 a. m. sailed in company with his Majesty's ship Boyne, and Hawk schooner.
7	8 12 8	82 83 82	17° 42″		7	ESE **	. .	cl.	The hospital ulcer, and gout, well; 2 feverish complaints, and 1 guinea worm added to the list; 11 in it. Some of the complaints returned from the hospital, worse than when they were sent.
8	8 12 8	82 83 82	17° 58″ R.		8	V ESE *	. .	cl.	Two bilious complaints added to the list; 13 in it. The feverish complaint added the 6th, is a bad remittent.
9	8 12 8	83 83 82	18° 05″		9	V **		c. cl.	The inflammation of the 1st, does duty; 12 in the list.
10	8 12 4 8	82 84 85 82	18° 10″		10	V *		c. cl.	An hæmoptosis added to the list; 13 in it.
11	8 12 8	83 84 83	18° 45″		11	V *	p. m. . . .	cl.	One of the feverish complaints of the 6th, and 1 of the 7th, well; 11 in the list.
12	8 12 4 8	82 83 85 83	19° 47″		12	V **		c. cl.	The headach of the 28th ult. and the 2 bilious complaints of the 8th, well; 8 in the list. Parted company with the Boyne, and lost sight of the Hawk.
13	8 12 8	83 84 83	20° 00″		13	V **		c. cl.	No alteration in the list.

Year, Months, and Days.	Hours.	Thermometer.	Latitude or different Parts.	Longitude made.	Moon's age.	Winds.	Rain or Dew	Appearances of the Atmosphere.	REMARKS, AND STATE OF THE SICK LIST.
1772 Julii 14	8 12 8	82 83 83	20° 04″		p. p. m	V E *		c. cl.	The other complaint of the 7th, and the guinea worm, well; 6 in the lift.
15	8 12 8	83 83 82	21° 14″		15	ESE *		c. cl.	No alteration in the lift. 6 p. m. took our departure from the Great Caicos.
16	8 12 8	82 83 82	23° 34	from the Great Caicos 00° 41″ E	16	ESE EbS **		cl.	Six in the lift.
17	8 12 8	82 83 83	24° 58″	01° 22″ E	17	f ESE t ENE *		cl.	No alteration in the lift.
18	8 12 8	8[illegible] 83 82	25° 25″	01° 36″ E	18	f ESE t *	a. m.	cl.	An inflammation added to the lift; 7 in it.
19	8 12 8	82 84 8[illegible]	26° 44″	02° 10″ E	19	V *	p. m.	cl.	The remittent of the 6th, well; 6 in the lift.
20	8 12 4 8	83 83 85 84	27° 40″	02° 58″ E	20	V *		cl.	No alteration in the lift. Scarce any wind.
21	8 12 8	83 84 83	27° 51″	03° 21″ E	21	V *		cl.	Six in the lift. Very hot, and fcarce any wind.
22	8 12 8	83 83 83	28° 12″	03° 51″ E	22	V *		cl.	One rheumatifm, and a diarrhœa added to the lift; 8 in it. The fame weather.
23	8 12 8	83 83 82	29° 02″	05° 12″ E	23	SSW *		c.	No alteration in the lift.
24	8 12 8	82 82 82	29° 42″	06° 23″ E	24	SSW *		c.	Eight in the lift.
25	8 12 8	83 83 83	29° 58″	07° 12″ E	25	*		c.	No alteration in the lift. Little or no wind, and very hot.
26	8 12 8	82 83 82	30° 43″	07° 42″ E	26	SE *		c.	Eight in the lift.

Year, Months, and Days.	Hours.	Thermometer.	Latitude or different parts.	Longitude made.	Moon's age.	Winds.	Rain or Dew.	Appearances of the Atmoſphere.	REMARKS, AND STATE OF THE SICK LIST.
1772 Julii 27	8 12 8	82 82 81	32° 08″	09° 00″ E	27	SE *		c.	No alteration in the liſt.
28	8 12 8	82 82 82	33° 14″	09° 52″ E	28	SE *		c.	The old hoſpital intermittent, and the Weaſel's man, returned to duty, 1 cough added to the liſt; 7 in it.
29	8 12 8	82 82 82	33° 30″	09° 52″ E	29	SE *		c.	No alteration in the liſt.
30	8 12 8	81 81 81	34° 07″	10° 32″ E	m. a. m.	SE *		c.	The cold of the 28th, returned to duty, 6 in the liſt.
31	8 12 8	80 81 80	34° 58″	11° 37″ E	2	SE —		c.	The inflammation of the 8th, well; 5 in the liſt, 1 Eryſipelas, 1 contuſion, 1 hæmoptoſis, 1 rheumatiſm, and 1 diarrhœa.
Aug. 1 Die Saturni	8 12 8	80 80 80	36° 07″	3° 44″ E from Gr. Caicos	3	SSW *		cl.	One feveriſh complaint added to the liſt; 6 in it.
2	8 12 8	80 80 79	37° 20″	16° 43″ E	4	f SWbS t NW **	...	cl.	The hæmoptoſis died, and 1 cough added to the liſt; 6 in it.
3	8 12 8	77 76 76	37° 48″	18° 57″ E	5	NNE *		cl. c.	The yeſterday's cough does duty, 5 in the liſt.
4	8 12 8	74 75 75	37°·20″	20° 51″ E	6	f NE t ENE *		cl. c.	The feveriſh complaint of the 1ſt, is a bad remittent fever. No alteration in the liſt.
5	8 12 8	74 74 75	37° 46″	21° 11″ E	7	f ESE t ENE *		cl. c.	The contuſion of the 2d ult. well; 4 in the liſt.
6	8 12 8	75 75 75	38° 32″	21° 24″ E	8	ESE **		cl. c.	One furuncle added to the liſt; 5 in it.
7	8 12 8	75 76 75	39° 11″	21° 33″ E	9	a. m. — p. m. NW *		cl. c.	No alteration in the liſt.
8	8 12 8	76 77 76	40° 03″	22° 35″ E	10	f NW t NWbN *		cl. c.	Five in the liſt.

Year, Months, and Days.	Hours.	Thermometer.	Latitude or different parts.	Longitude made.	Moon's age.	Winds.	Rain or Dew.	Appearances of the Atmosphere.	REMARKS, AND STATE OF THE SICK LIST.
1772 Aug. 9	8 12 4 8	76 76 78 76	40° 20″	23° 18″ E	11	f SbE t WSW —		c. cl.	No alteration in the liſt.
10	8 12 4 8	74 75 77 76	41° 00″	26° 12″ E	12	f SbE t WSW p. m. **		c. cl.	The furuncle of the 6th, well; 2 with feveriſh ſymptoms added to the liſt; 6 in it.
11	8 12 8	76 75 74	41° 44″	29° 21″ E	13	SW **	. . .	cl.	The eryſipelas, and the diarrhœa of the 22d, well; 1 feveriſh complaint, and 1 contuſion added to the liſt; 6 in it.
12	8 12 8	73 71 71	42° 14″	32° 47″ E	14	NW **		cl.	Yeſterday's contuſion well; n the liſt.
13	8 12 8	69 70 72	42° 24″	35° 05″ E	p. . a. m.	a. m. NW p.m WSW **		cl. c.	The remitting fever died, 4 in the liſt.
14	8 12 8	73 73 70	43° 09″	38° 10″ E	16	f SWbW t WNW **		cl.	Two with feveriſh ſymptoms of the 10th, well 1 feveriſh complaint, and 1 cough added to the liſt; 4 in it.
15	8 12 4 8	68 69 71 69	43° 41″	40° 17″ E	17	NbE ENE *		cl. c.	One with feveriſh ſymptoms added to the liſt; 5 in it.
16	8 12 8	68 68 68	43° 46″	42° 37″ E	18	NbE ENE *		c. cl.	Yeſterday's, and the feveriſh complaint of the 11th, well; 1 with feveriſh ſymptoms added to the liſt; 4 in it.
17	8 12 8	68 68 70	43° 37″	44° 21″ E	19	NbE ENE **		c. cl.	The complaints of the 14th, and yeſterday's, well; 1 headach, and a rheumatiſm, added to the liſt; 3 in it.
18	8 12 4 8	69 67 72 71	43° 43″	45° 15″ E	20	f WNW t NW **		cl.	Two with feveriſh ſymptoms; and 1 contuſion added to the liſt; 6 in it.
19	8 12 8	70 69 67	45° 01″	47° 54″	21	WNW NE ***	. . .	cl.	The rheumatiſm of the 17th, well; and an inflammation added to the liſt; 6 in it
20	8 12 8	65 64 63	45° 18″	49° 20″ E	22	f NbE t NW **		cl.	No alteration in the liſt.

Year, Months, and Days.	Hours.	Thermometer	Latitude or different parts.	Longitude made.	Moon's Age	Winds.	Rain and Dew.	Appearances of the Atmosphere.	REMARKS, AND STATE OF THE SICK LIST.
1772 Aug. 21	8 12 8	63 63 64	46° 40″	51° 35″ E	23	NW ***		c. cl.	One of the feverish complaints of the 18th, well; in the list.
22	8 12 8	61 60 59	48° 48″	54° 33″ E	24	f W t WSW ****	. . .	cl.	One with feverish symptoms added to the list; 6 in it.
23	8 12 4 8	59 59 63 61	49° 35″	60° 09″ E	25	f NW t WSW ***	. .	cl.	The headach of the 17th, the contusion of the 18th, and the inflammation of the 19th, well; 1 headach added to the list; 4 in it.
24	8 12 4 8	61 62 65 63	49° 34″	From the Great Caieos 64° 51″ E	26	f WSW t WNW ***		cl.	The feverish complaint of the 22d, and yesterday's headach well; 2 in the list.
25	8 12 8	61 64 62	49° 57″ Lizzard		27	f WSW t NW***		cl.	No alteration in the list. A. m. made the lizzard.
26	8 12 8	61	M Spithead		28	f WSW t NW **		c.	The other feverish complaint of the 8th, well; the only complaint in the list, is a rheumatism, an old man, who likewise has a suffusion in one of his eyes; and is to be sent to the hospital with the ulcers. Anchor'd at noon.

END OF THE FIRST VOYAGE.

CHAPTER II.

THE DIARY OF THE WEATHER AND STATE OF THE SICK LIST, BETWEEN THE 30th OF NOVEMBER 1772, AND THE 24th OF AUGUST 1773.

Year, Months, and Days.	Hours.	Thermometer.	Latitude or different parts.	Longitude made.	Moon's age.	Winds.	Rain or Dew.	Appearances of the Atmosphere.	REMARKS, AND STATE OF THE SICK LIST.
1772 Nov. 30 Die Lunæ			Cowes		6	E S **	. .	h. cl.	Seven in the list. 3 colds with feverish symptoms, 1 old intermittent, 1 fractured clavicle, 1 scald, and 1 contusion. M. Sailed from Spithead, and anchor'd at Cowes at 2 p. m.
Dec. 1					7	SSW **	.	h. cl.	One cough, 1 wound, and 1 contusion added to the list; 10 in it.
2	12 8	58 65 f			8	f SE t ESE **		cl.	Yesterday's cough does duty; 9 in the list. All the complaints are the consequence of intemperance.
3	8 12 8	61 f 65 f 65 f	Off Plymouth		9	f ENE t SE **		h.	One cold of the 30th, well; and a quinsey added to the list; 9 in it. His Majesty's Sloop Dispatch, joined us company p. m.
4	8 12 8	61 f 62 f 67 f	48° 33″ R.	from the Ram head 02° 11″ W	10	SE ***		h.	One fever, 1 cough, and 1 ulcer, added to the list, 12 in it.
5	8 12 8	62 f 64 f 67 f	47° 05″	05° 04″ W	11	f E t ESE **		h.	The contusion of the 1st, and the quinsey of the 3d, well; 3 colds with feverish complaints added to the list; 13 in it.
6	8 12 8	60 f 60 f 67 f	47° 50″	06° 26″ W	12	W NW **		cl.	The contusion of the 30th, 1 of the colds, and 2 of yesterday's complaints, well; 9 in the list. The fever of the 4th is a remittent.
7	8 12 8	55 55 55	44° 28″	07° 57″ W	13	f NNW t NE **		cl.	The other cold of the 30th ult. well; 8 in the list
8	8 12 8	61 f 61 f 65 f	41° 52″	09° 51″ W	14	f NNW t NE **		c. cl.	The cough of the 4th, well; 7 in the list.
9	8 12 8	62 64 67	39° 26″	10° 50″ W	15	NE **		c.	No alteration in the list.
10	8 12 8	64 67 70	37° 14″	11° 08″ W	16 P. p. m.	NNE **		c.	The wound of the 1st, and the ulcer of the 4th, well; 5 in it.
11	8 12 8	64 67 69	35° 20″	11° 20″ W	17	f NNE t NE *		cl.	One lame, and 1 with feverish symptoms added to the list; 7 in it.
12	8 2 8	65 66 66	33° 34″	11° 40″ W	18	f NNE t ENE **		cl.	No alteration in the list.

Year, Months, and Days.	Hours.	Thermometer.	Latitude or different parts.	Longitude made.	Moon's age.	Winds.	Rain or Dew.	Appearances of the Atmosphere.	REMARKS, AND STATE OF THE SICK LIST
1772 Dec. 13	8 12 8	64 f 66 f 70 f	Madeira	in 17° 20″ W Porto Sancto	19	NE *		cl.	The complaints of the 11th, well; 5 in the list: 5 p. m anchored with the Dispatch in Foncheall Bay.
14	8 12 8	67 f 70 f 68 f		Madeira in 18° 11″ W	20	Sb & lb *		c.	The scald, the old intermittent, and the fractured clavicle of the 30th ult. well; 2 in the list.
15	8 12 8	66 f 68 f 67	32° 32″		21	f ENE t EbS **		c.	A swelled parotid added to the list; 3 in it. Sailed with the Dispatch at 11 a. m.
16	8 12 8	66 f 69 f 71 f	30° 25″		22	f ENE t EbS **		c.	No alteration in the list.
17	8 12 8	67 f 69 f 72 f	28° 47″	From Maderia 00° 45″ E	23	f ENE t EbS *		c.	One cough, 1 sore throat, 1 sickness at stomach and 1 with eruptions, added to the list; 7 in it. Began serving spruce beer to the ship's company. Teneriffe.
18	8 12 8	71 f 72 f 69 f	Teneriffe		24	f ENE t EbS *		c.	The sickness at stomach added yesterday, well; 1 cold, suppressed perspiration, added to the list 7 in it. 9 a. m. anchor'd in St. Cruze Road.
19	8 12 8	70 69 71			25	Sb & lb **		c.	The cough of the 17th, well; 6 in the list.
20	8 12 8	69 71 69			26	Sb & lb **		c.	No alteration in the list. His Majesty's transport Endeavour came in, she had 2 lieutenants, &c. on board.
21	8 12 8	70 71 71			27	Sb & lb *		c.	The remittent of the 4th, and 1 of the feverish complaints of the 5th, well; 4 in the lift.
22	8 12 8	69 70 69			28	Sb & lb *		c.	The complaint with eruptions of the 17th, and the cold of the 18th, well; 2 in the list. On the tops of the mountains there is frost in the night.
23	8 12 8	68 70 69			29	Sb & lb *		c.	No alteration in the list
24	8 12 8	71 70 70			m. a. m.	Sb & lb *		c.	Two in the list.
25	8 12 8	70 68 70	28° 05″		2	NE *		c.	Sailed with the Dispatch, and Endeavour, at 1 a. m.

Year, Months, and Days.	Hours.	Thermometer.	Latitude or different Parts.	Longitude made.	Moon's age.	Winds.	Rain or Dew.	Appearances of the Atmosphere.	REMARKS, AND STATE OF THE SICK LIST.
1772 Dec. 26	8 12 8	70 70 69	26° 05″	00° 05″ W from the Pick	3	f E t ESE **		c. cl.	No alteration in the list. The Endeavour parted company in the night.
27	8 12 8	67 67 67	23° 05″	00° 16″ W	4	E *	✣	c.	One added to the list, with a sickness at stomach; 2 in it.
28	8 12 8	65 65 71 f.	20° 46″ Cape Blancho	00° 15″ W	5	f E t NNE *	✣	c. cl.	No alteration in the list. Off the coast of Barbary.
29	8 12 8	68 68 69	19° 05″	00° 07″ W	6	f ENE t ESE *	✣	c. cl.	The complaint of the 27th, well; 2 in the list.
30	8 12 8	68 69 68	18° 05″	00° 43″ E	7	NE*	✣	c. cl.	The parotid of the 15th, well; 1 Guinea worm who lately came from a *Guinea* ship, added to the list; 2 in it.
31	8 12 8	68 68 69	16° 34″	00° 38″ E	8	NE *	✣	a. m. h.	No alteration in the list. At 5 p. m. anchor'd off Senegal Fort with the Dispatch. A very great surf on the Beach.
1773 Jan. 1 Die Veneris	8 12 8	69 69 71	Senegal		9	NE **	✣	h.	Two lame complaints added to the list; 4 in it. The garrison has been very sickly, and lost a number of men. A Canoe came off.
2	8 12 8	70 71 72			10	NE *	✣	c.	One sore throat, 1 Guinea worm, and yesterday's complaints in the list. The Dispatch dropped down and anchored off the bar.
3	8 12 8	71 71 71			11	NE *	✣	h. p. m.	One abscess, and 1 lame complaint, added to the list; 6 in it. No boat can land yet.
4	8 12 8	72 72 72			12	NE *	✣	h.	The two lame complaints of the 1st, and yesterday's, well; 2 in the list. P. m. joined the Dispatch, and sailed together.
5	8 12 8	73 72 73	15° 29″	from Senegal Fort. 00° 43″ W	13	NbE*	✣	cl.	One sore throat added to the list; 3 in it.
6	8 12 8	73 73 73	15° 26″	02° 37″ W	14	NbE *	✣	cl.	No alteration in the list.
7	8 12 8	73 73 73	15° 26″	04° 26″ W	15	NbE **		cl.	The sore throat of the 5th, well; 2 in the list.

Year, Months, and Days.	Hours.	Thermometer.	Latitude or different Parts.	Longitude made.	Moon's age.	Winds.	Rain or Dew.	Appearances of the Atmosphere.	REMARKS, AND STATE OF THE SICK LIST.
1773 Jan. 8	8 12 8	73 73 74	15° 05″		p. p. m.	NNE **		c.	No alteration in the lift. A gouty complaint but not in it. At 1 p. m. anchor'd at Maijo one of the Cape de Verde ifland's, it is very barren and hilly. The inhabitants are all black, and employed in making falt; and the little ftock which they have chiefly, comes from St. Jago the moft fertile of thefe iflands.
9	8 12 8	74 73 74	Maijo		17	NNE **		c.	Two in the lift.
10	8 12 8	73 73 74			18	NNE *		cl.	Two with feverifh complaints added to the lift; 4 in it. Got a few lean bullocks for the fhip's company. They have bought fome goats, and Hogs, &c.
11	8 12 8	72 72 73	St. Jago		19	NNE		cl.	One of yefterday's complaints, well; 3 in the lift. Sailed at 4 a. m. and anchor'd at 8 a. m. with the Difpatch in Praija Bay, St. Jago.
12	8 12 8	72 73 73			20	NNE **		c. cl.	No alteration in the lift. Sailed with the Difpatch at 5 p. m. we got very little ftock.
13	8 12 8	72 73 73	13° 48″	from Praija Bay 01° 45″ E	21	NE **	✣	cl.	No alteration in the lift.
14	8 12 8	73 74 74	12° 15″	03° 43″ E	22	NE **	✣	cl.	Three in the lift. A number of bilious complaints on board the Difpatch.
15	8 12 8	75 74 74	11° 00″	05° 45″ E	23	NE. *	✣	cl.	One of the feverifh complaints of the 10th, well; 1 ftrain added to the lift; 3 in it. After confulting the Captain, I made a quarter cafk of wine into a tincture of bark. *Vid Poftfcript.*
16	8 12 8	74 76 78	10° 10″	06° 47″ E	24	*	✣	h.	Yefterday's complaint does duty; 2 in the lift.
17	8 12 8	77 77 78	09° 33″	07° 13″ E	25	—	✣	h.	No alteration in the lift, Very fultry.
18	8 12 4 8	78 79 81 105 80	09° 07″	07° 27″ E	26	*	✣	c.	The Guinea worm of the 24th ult. well; 1 in the lift. Very hot. In ten minutes the thermometer rofe in the Sun's rays, 24 degrees.
19	8 12 4 8	80 81 82 81	09° 12″	08° 10″ E	27	N *		h.	No alteration in the lift. Very hazy, notwithftanding the fun fhines

Year, Months, and Days.	Hours.	Thermometer.	Latitude or different parts.	Longitude made.	Moon's age	Winds.	Rain or Dew.	Appearances of the Atmoſphere.	REMARKS, AND STATE OF THE SICK LIST.
20	8 12 4 8	81 81 83 82	08° 43″	09° 19″ E	28	N. NE*	✣	h.	One ſickneſs at ſtomach added to the liſt; 2 in it. p. m. anchored off Sierra Leon River, with the Diſpatch. Very hot.
21	8 12 8	82 81 81	Sierra Leon.		29	lb.	✣	h.	Yeſterday's complaint well; 1 fever added to the liſt. At 3 p. m. anchor'd in Sierra Leon River. Some merchant ſhips, whoſe men have been very ſickly, lying here.
22	8 12 4 8	79 80 82 81			m. p. m	Sb & lb	✣	h.	No alteration in the liſt. Gave five ounces of the tincture of bark, to every man before they were ſent aſhore in the morning on duty; and they were ſtrictly forbid having any communication with the merchantmen's people. The ſame method was obſerved on board of the Diſpatch, from having it recommended there.
23	8 12 8	80 81 81			1	Sb & lb	✣	h.	One inflammation added to the liſt; 3 in it. Gave the tincture of bark to the ſhorers. They all ſleep on board.
24	8 12 8	79 80 81			2	Sb & lb	✣	h.	The Guinea worm complaint diſcharged, the 18th relapſed; 1 opthalmia, and 2 with feveriſh ſymptoms added to the liſt; 7 in it. No ſhore duty, being Sunday
25	8 12 8	80 80 81			3	Sb & lb	✣	h.	No alteration in the liſt. Gave the tincture of bark to the ſhorers; an old man came on board that we left here laſt year on board of a ſhip.
26	8 12 8	80 81 81			4	Sb & lb	✣	h.	One of the feveriſh complaints of the 24th, well; 6 in the liſt, gave the ſhorers the tincture of bark.
27	8 12 8	80 81 81			5	Sb & lb	✣	h.	One drunken complaint added to the liſt; 7 in it. The men get New England rum from the blacks. Adminiſtered the tincture as uſual.
28	8 12 4 8	78 80 82 81			6	Sb & lb	✣	h.	The other feveriſh complaint of the 24th, well; 1 bilious, and 1 lame complaints added to the liſt; 8 in it. Gave the tincture to the ſhorers—the wooding, and watering parties, and boat's crews.
29	8 12 4 8	79 80 82 81			7	Sb & lb	✣	h.	The opthalmia of the 24th, and yeſterday's bilious complaints well; 1 contuſion added to the liſt; Repeated the tincture of bark.
30	8 12 8	79 81 81			8	Sb & lb	✣	h.	One inflammation added to the liſt; 8 in it. Shore duty over. Four ounces of the tincture was the doſe given on board of the Diſpatch.
31	8 12 8	81 81 81			9	f NNW t NW	✣	h.	The drunken complaint of the 27th, the lame of the 28th, and the contuſion of the 29th, well; 2 with ſickneſs at ſtomach; and an abſceſs added to the liſt.

Year, Months, and Days.	Hours.	Thermometer.	Latitude or different parts.	Longitude made.	Moon's age.	Winds.	Rain or Dew.	Appearances of the Atmosphere	REMARKS, AND STATE OF THE SICK LIST.
1773 Feb. 1 Die Lunæ	8 12 4 8	81 81 82 81	08° 15″		10	f NNW t NW *		h.	Yesterday's ficknefs's at ftomach, well; 1 added to the lift with gripes—Thofe complaints proceed from eating unripe plantings, bananas, and fifh; and 1 contufion, 8 in the lift; 2 inflammations, 1 with gripes, 1 remittent, 1 fore throat; and 3 lame complaints.
2	8 12 4 8	81 81 82 81	07° 40″	from Cape Sierra Leon 00° 35″ W	11	V *	❖	h.	No alteration in the lift. The Difpatch's men are ftill afflicted with bilious complaints.
3	8 12 8	80 78 79	07° 13″	00° 15″ W	12	V *	. ❖	h. cl.	The Guinea worm of the 24th ult. and contufion of the 1ft well; 6 in the lift.
4	8 12 8	80 79 79	06° 51″	00° 08″ E	13	p. m. ※	. ❖	h. cl.	The fever; the inflammation of the 30th ult. and the griped complaint of the 1ft, well; 3 in the lift.
5	8 12 8	80 79 80	06° 40″	01° 12″ E	14	N *	. ❖	h. cl.	The abfcefs of the 31ft ult. well; 2 in the lift. No perfon on board finds himfelf refrefhed from fleep.
6	8 12 8	80 80 79	05° 46″	00° 48″ E	15	V *	. ❖	h. cl.	No alteration in the lift. Very dull weather, which depreffes every one's fpirits, 10 men in the Difpatch's fick lift.
7	8 12 8	79 79 79	04° 26″	01° 18″ E	p. a. m.	V *	❖	h. cl.	Two in the lift ftill. The fame kind of weather yet; and no perfon is refrefhed from his fleep.
8	8 12 8	79 79 79	04° 56″	01° 57″ E	17	V *	❖	h.	One with eruptions added to the lift; 3 in it. Every thing amazingly damp and mouldy on board. Wood opens at the joints, and fhrinks greatly, and iron rufts.
9	8 12 8	78 80 81	04° 30″	02° 37″ E	18	V *	❖	h.	One who was afhore fifhing at Sierra Leon, added to the lift with feverifh fymptoms; 4 in it. The fifhermen were not allowed the tincture.
10	8 12 8	79 80 79	04° 16″	from Cape Palmas 00° 33″ E	19	V *	❖	h.	One inflammation added to the lift; 5 in it.
11	8 12 8	76 75 76	04° 32″	01° 40″ E	20	V **	. . . ❖	h. cl.	No alteration in the lift. Very cold and difagreeable weather.
12	8 12 4 8	76 76 80 79	05° 03″	03° 09″ E	21	N *	❖	h. cl.	The complaint of the 9th, well; 4 in the lift. Our fails quite black with mildew. The dews are very heavy.

Year, Months, and Days.	Hours.	Thermometer	Latitude or different parts.	Longitude made.	Moon's Age	Winds.	Rain and Dew.	Appearances of the Atmosphere.	REMARKS, AND STATE OF THE SICK LIST.
1773 Feb. 13	8 12 4 8	78 79 82 80	05° 16″	from Cape Le Hou 00° 58″ E	22	N *	✣	h. cl.	No alteration in the lift. Loft fight of the Difpatch.
14	8 12 4 8	80 80 82 80	04° 05″ Appaloni		23	N **	✣	cl.	The inflammation of the 10th, well; 3 in the lift. The Difpatch in fight. Anchor'd m. at Appalonia, failed at 4 p. m. and anchor'd at 8 p. m. in the offing.
15	8 12 8	81 80 80	Axim		24	V *	✣	cl. c.	The complaint of the 8th, well; 1 rheumatifm added to the lift; 3 in it. Sailed at 8 a. m. and anchor'd at 1 p. m. at Axim, a Dutch fettlement, with an intention to water the fhip; but they have none, it is fo long fince they had rain. The Difpatch out of fight.
16	8 12 8	81 81 81			25	Sb & lb		cl. c.	No alteration in the lift. The Difpatch joined, and left us again; 10 in their lift.
17	8 12 8	78 80 80	05° 00″ Cape Coaft		26	Sb & lb	✣	cl. c.	Three in the lift yet. At 4 p. m. anchor'd at Cape Coaft.
18	8 12 8	80 82 82			27	✣	. . .	cl.	No alteration in the lift. The Difpatch joined us, none of their people dangeroufly ill.
19	8 12 8	79 80 80			28	✣	. . . ✣	cl.	The inflammation of the 23d ult. well; 2 in the lift. The men can get no frefh ftock, fruit nor vegetables to buy.
20	8 12 8	78 81 80			29	Sb & lb	. ✣	cl.	One with feverifh fymptoms added to the lift; 3 in it. The waterers here and boat's crew, take the tincture. It is Pond water we get.
21	8 12 8	78 81 80			m. m.	Sb & lb	✣	cl.	No alteration in the lift. Gave the waterers the tincture. The water has no bad tafte though thick; it is well ftrained and intended for the live ftock, and boiling only. There was quick lime thrown into the Pond before we took any out of it. The men get fpirits from the blacks.
22	8 12 4 8	80 81 82 81			2	Sb & lb		cl. c.	The rheumatifm of the 15th, and the feverifh of the 20th, well; 1 in the fick lift. Gave the waterers the tincture. The feverifh complaint returned to duty to-day, was a wooder at Sierra Leon.
23	8 12 8	82 82 82			3	Sb & lb	✣	cl. c.	A drunken cook added to the lift, with feverifh fymptoms; 2 in it. 6 in the Difpatch's lift. All the people on the coaft healthy.

Year, Months, and Days.	Hours.	Thermometer.	Latitude or different Parts.	Longitude made.	Moon's age.	Winds.	Rain or Dew.	Appearances of the Atmosphere.	REMARKS, AND STATE OF THE SICK LIST.
1773 Feb. 24	8 12 8	80 82 79			4	p. m. ※	. . .	cl.	One with feverish symptoms, and 1 headach added to the list; 4 in it. Sailed in the evening, and left the Dispatch to run down to Accra. Always cold in the time of the Tornado's.
25	8 12 8	79 80 81	04° 55″		5	Sb & lb		h.	No alteration in the list. We got a very small supply at Cape Coast, either of stock, fruit, or vegetables, and none any where else on the coast.
26	8 12 4 8	81 81 83 82	04° 40″		6	Sb & lb		h.	One headach, and 1 rheumatism added to the list; 6 in it. These complaints are the consequence of the new rum which they got from the Negroes, or free black people.
27	8 12 4 8	82 82 83 82	04° 57		7	WSW *		h.	No alteration in the list.
28	8 12 4 8	82 82 83 82	04° 24″	from Cape Appalonia 00° 09″ E	8	WSW *		h.	The headach of the 24th well; the headach of the 26th, has a sore throat, which seems to be venereal; 5 in the list.
Martii 1 Die Lunæ	8 12 8	82 83 82	03° 28″	00° 56″ E	9	WSW *		h.	The feverish of the 23d, and the feverish complaints of the 24th well, 1 suppressed perspiration, or cold, added to the list; 4 in it. One old sore throat, 1 headach, 1 rheumatism, and this day's complaint.
2	8 12 4 8	81 82 84 82	02° 41″	01° 22″ E	10	f S t SWbS **	. .	h. cl.	One added to the list, with a sickness at stomach; 5 in it.
3	8 12 8	82 82 82	02° 24″	00° 58″ E	11	V *	.	h. cl.	The rheumatism of the 26th ult, and the cold of the 1st well; 3 in the list.
4	8 12 4 8	82 82 83 82	02° 11″	01° 03″ E	12	V *		h. cl.	No alteration in the list.
5	8 12 4 8	83 83 84 83	02° 09″	00° 22″ E	13	f SbW t SWbW *		h. cl.	The old man that came on board at Sierra Leon, complained of a sickness at stomach, and a feverish complaint added to the list; 5 in it.
6	8 12 8	83 83 83	02° 18″	00° 40″ E	14	SbW *		h.	A great many fish playing about the ship. No alteration in the list.

P

Year, Months, and Days.	Hours.	Thermometer.	Latitude or different parts.	Longitude made.	Moon's age.	Winds.	Rain or Dew.	Appearances of the Atmosphere.	REMARKS, AND STATE OF THE SICK LIST.
1773. March 7	8 12 8	83 83 83	02° 40″	02° 13″ W	15	S SbW t SWbS *		h	The complaints of the 5th, well; 3 in the lift. The complaint of the 2d has a cough.
8	8 12 4 8	82 83 84 83	02° 50″	03° 10″ W	p. p. m.	SbW SSW *		h.	No alteration in the lift. The fpruce beer is all expended, and wine began to be ferved to the fhip's company.
9	8 12 4 8	83 83 84 83	02° 54″	04° 27″ W	17	SbW SSW *	❖	h.	One fore throat added to the lift; 4 in it.
10	8 12 8	83 83 83	02° 54″ R.	04° 53″ W	18	f W t SSW *	. . .	cl. t.	No alteration in the lift. Sultry difagreeable weather.
11	8 12 8	82 83 82	02° 23″	04° 56″ W	19	V *	❖	cl.	One lame complaint added to the lift; 5 in it.
12	8 12 8	82 83 82	02° 29″	05° 15″ W from Cape Appalonia	20	SW p. m **	❖	cl. c.	An incifion added to the lift; 6 in it.
13	8 12 8	83 83 83	03° 12″	06° 55″ W	21	SW **	❖	cl. c.	The fore throat of the 9th, well; 5 in the lift.
14	8 12 8	83 84 83	04° 07″	08° 44″ W	22	V *	. . . .	cl. t. l.	No alteration in the lift.
15	8 12 8	83 83 83	04° 13″	08° 58″ W	23	V *	. . . .	cl. t. l.	Five in the lift. Exceeding bad weather, and very little wind.
16	8 12 4 8	83 82 79 81	04° 09′	09° 02′ W	24	V ***	. . . .	cl. t. l.	One rheumatick complaint added to the lift; 6 in it. The old fore throat is a fcorbutick rheumatifm. No wind, but in fqualls.
1	8 12 8	82 83 8[illegible]	04° 31″	10° 02″ W	25	V ***	. .	cl. h.	The complaint of the 2d, well; 5 in the lift. Almoft calm except during the fqualls.
18	8 2	82 79 80	04° 54″	10° 28″ W	26	V ***	. . . .	cl. t. l.	The old fore throat returned to duty, 4 in the lift. The men are often expofed to the rains.

Year, Months, and Days.	Hour.	Thermometer.	Latitude or different parts.	Longitude made.	Moon's age.	Winds.	Rain or Dew.	Appearances of the Atmoſphere.	REMARKS, AND STATE OF THE SICK LIST.
1773 Martii 19	8 12 8	81 79 79	05° 10″	10 50″ W	27	V *	. . . .	cl. t. l.	No alteration in the liſt, nor weather.
20	8 12 8	80 80 79	04° 58″	11° 01″ W	28	V *	. . . .	cl. t. l.	Four in the liſt. No perſon on board thinks himſelf at all refreſhed from his ſleep.
21	8 12 8	80 81 80	04° 44″	11° 12″ W	29	V *	. . .	cl.	One nephritick complaint, and 1 with eruptions, added to the liſt; 6 in it.
22	8 12 8	81 82 81	04° 23″	11° 18″ W	30	V * .	. .	cl. t. l.	No alteration in the liſt.
23	8 12 8	82 83 80	04° 53″	11° 32″ W	n. m. a. m.	V ***	. . . .	cl. t. l.	The rheumatick complaint of the 16th, well; wind, only in the ſqualls.
24	8 12 8	82 82 82	05° 25″	12° 13″ W	2	V ***	. .	cl. t. l.	The inciſion of the 12th, well; 4 in the liſt.
25	8 12 8	80 80 81	05° 33″	12° 53″ W	3	ENE *	. . .	cl. h.	No alteration in the liſt.
26	8 12 8	83 82 82	05° 33″	13° 05″ W	4	V *	. .	cl. h.	The nephritick complaint of the 21ſt, well; 3 in the liſt.
27	8 12 8	82 82 80	05° 39″ R.	13° 15″ W	5	V *	.	cl. h.	No alteration in the liſt.
28	8 12 8	80 78 80	05° 49″	13° 33″ W	6	V *	. . . .	cl. h.	Three in the liſt. Very diſagreeable weather.
29	8 12 8	82 82 82	05° 46″	13° 39″ W	7	NbW *		c.	An aſthmatick complaint added to the liſt; 4 in it.
30	8 12 8	82 81 78	05° 29″	14° 29″ W	8	SE p. m. ***	. . . .	cl t. l.	One with feveriſh ſymptoms, and 1 ſickneſs at ſtomach, added to the liſt; 6 in it. Very cold during the ſquall.
31	8 12 8	81 81 81	05° 44″	14° 50″ W	9	V *		cl.	The headach of the 26th ult. well; 5 in the liſt. 1 remittent, 1 nauſea, 1 lame, 1 with eruptions, and 1 aſthmatick complaint.

Year, Months, and Days.	Hours.	Thermometer	Latitude or different parts.	Longitude made.	Moon's Age	Winds.	Rain and Dew.	Appearances of the Atmosphere.	REMARKS, AND STATE OF THE SICK LIST.
1773 Die Jovis April. 1	8 12 8	80 81 80	05° 23″	15°22″ W	10	f NbW t NW		cl.	No alteration in the list. The feverish complaint of the 30th, is the remittent fever.
2	8 12 8	80 80 80	04° 54″	16°06″ W	11	NW *		cl.	The complaint with eruptions of the 21st ult. well; 4 in the list.
3	8 12 8	80 79 80	04° 50″	16°42″ W	12	V a. m. p. m. N *	. . .	cl.	No alteration in the list.
4	8 12 8	80 80 80	04° 30″	18°20″ W	13	NbE W *	.	cl.	The sickness at stomach of the 30th ult. well; 1 dry belly-ach added to the list; 4 in it.
5	8 12 8	81 81 81	03° 23″	from Cape Appalonia 19°33″ W	14	f N t NNE *		c.	No alteration in the list.
6	8 12 8	81 80 79	03° 29″	20°24″ W	15	NNE *	.	c. cl.	The dry belly ach of the 4th, well; 3 in the list.
7	8 12 8	80 80 79	03° 28″	21°14″ W	p. a. m.	NNE **		c.	The lame complaint of the 11th ult. well; 1 ulcer added to the list; 3 in it. Pleasant weather.
8	8 12 8	80 80 79	03° 57″	23°05″ W	17	NNE **		cl.	No alteratton in the list.
9	8 12 8	80 80 78	04° 23″	25°06″ W	18	NNE **		cl. c.	One with feverish symptoms added to the list; 4 in it.
10	8 12 8	80 80 79	04° 44″	26°48″ W	19	NNE **		cl. c.	No alteration in the list.
11	8 12 8	80 80 79	05° 09″	28°23″ W	20	NNE NEbN **		cl. c.	Four in the list. The feverish complaint added to the list the 9th is a remitting fever.
12	8 12 8	79 80 79	05° 42″	30°34″ W	21	NEbE **		cl.	No alteration in the list.
13	8 12 8	80 80 79	06° 41″	32° 39″ W	22	NE **		cl.	One feverish complaint added to the list; 5 in it.

Year, Months, and Days.	Hours.	Thermometer.	Latitude of different Parts.	Longitude made.	Moon's age.	Winds.	Rain or Dew.	Appearance of the Atmoſphere.	REMARKS, AND STATE OF THE SICK LIST.
1773 Aprilis 14	8 12 8	79 79 77	07° 45″	35° 10″ W	23	NE **		cl.	he remittent fever of the 30th ult well; 4 the liſt.
15	8 12 8	78 77 77	08° 51″	37° 03″ W	24	NE **	.	cl.	One with feveriſh ſymptoms added to the liſt; 5 in it. Very cold.
16	8 12 8	78 78 77	09° 51″	39° 21″ W	25	NEbE **		cl.	The old ſcorbutick rheumatiſm added to the liſt; 6 in it.
17	8 12 8	77 77 76	10° 56″	41° 48″ W	26	ENE **		cl.	The complaint of the 13th well; and an opthalmia added to the liſt; 6 in it.
18	8 12 8	77 77 76	12° 11″	44° 08″ W	27	ENE **		cl.	The remitting fever of the 9th well; and 1 lumbago added to the liſt; 6 in it. The feveriſh complaint of the 15th, is a bad remitting fever.
19	8 12 8	78 77 77	13° 20″	46° 15″ W	28	ENE **	.	cl.	One headach, and 2 with the rheumatiſm added to the liſt; 9 in it.
20	8 12 8	76 76 76	14° 30″	48° 26″ W	29	V *		cl.	No alteration in the liſt.
21	8 12 8	75 76 76	15° 35″	50° 10″ W	m. p. m	V *	.	cl.	Nine in the liſt. Very cold.
22	8 12 8	77 76 76	16° 04″	52° 11″ W	1	ENE **		cl.	The headach of the 19th, well; and 1 feveriſh complaint added to the liſt; 9 in it.
23	8 12 8	78 77 76	16° 18″	54° 24″ W	2	ENE E **		cl. c.	No alteration in the liſt.
24	8 12 8	79 77 77	16° 22″	56° 23″ W	3	EbN **		c.	Nine in the liſt. Some ulcers who are not in the liſt. The ſun is right a ſtern a. m. which makes the Thermometer higheſt then, though his rays do not ſhine upon it.
25	8 12 8	80 77 78	16° 26″	58° 06″ W	4	V **		c.	One of the rheumatiſms of the 19th, and the feveriſh complaint of the 22d well; 7 in the liſt.
26	8 12 8	79 78 78	16° 24″		5	V *		c.	No alteration in the liſt. The ulcers are become ſcorbutick—The ſhip's reckoning is out.

O

Year, Months, and Days.	Hours.	Thermometer	Latitude or different parts.	Longitude made.	Moon's Age	Winds.	Rain and Dew.	Appearances of the Atmosphere.	REMARKS, AND STATE OF THE SICK LIST.
1773 Aprilis 27	8 12 8	78 78 79	16° 32″		6	V *		c.	No alteration in the list. Scorbutick symptoms appear amongst the sick.
28	8 12 8	79 79 79	m Antigua		7	V *		c.	Seven in the list. Anchor'd at noon in English harbour. Admiral Parry commands; 4 of His Majesty's ships in it.
29	8 12 8	79 81 80			8	*		c.	Two headachs with a nausea, 1 subject to it, and 1 scorbutick ulcer added to the list; 10 in it. They received great damage both on board and ashore, by a late hurricane. No vegetables.
30	8 12 8	79 80 78			9	Sb & lb		c.	The ulcer of the 7th, the opthalmia of the 17th, and 1 of yesterday's headachs, the old one well; 7 in the list. 1 asthma, 1 scorbutick rheumatism, 2 rheumatisms, 1 remitting fever, 1 headach, and 1 ulcer. We lye in a part of the harbour called Freeman's bay.
Maii 1 Die Saturni	8 12 8	78 78 79			10	Sb & lb		c.	The lumbago or rheumatism of the 18th ult. well; 6 in the list. P. m. sailed. The men drunk with new rum.
2	8 12 8	80 81 80	St. Christophers		11	NE **		c. cl.	No alteration in the sick list. They suffered greatly here too by the hurricane. No fresh provisions nor vegetables here either.
3	8 12 8	80 81 81			12	NE **	. .	cl.	One feverish complaint added to the list; 7 in it. This island produces plenty of vegetables commonly.
4	8 12 8	81 80 81	17° 17″		13	NE **		cl.	No alteration in the list. Sailed at 8 a. m.
5	8 12 8	81 80 79	17° 18″	from St. Christophers 02° 34″ W	14	NE EbN *		cl.	The other headach of the 29th, well; and the old man who came on board at Sierra Leon, added to the list; 7 in it.
6	8 12 8	80 80 80	17° 23″	04° 23″ W	p. p. m.	NE EbN *		c. cl.	The remitting fever of the 15th, the other rheumatism of the 19th ult. the feverish complain of the 3d, and yesterday's complaint well. 2 nauseas from drunkenness, and 1 with eruptions added to the list; 6 in it.
7	8 12 8	81 80 80	17° 18″	05° 59″ W	16	NE EbN *		c.	No alteration in the list.
8	8 12 8	81 81 81	17° 28″	06° 53″ W	17	NE EbN *		c. cl.	One of the nauseas of the 6th, well; 5 in the list

Year, Months, and Days.	Hours.	Thermometer.	Latitude or different parts.	Longitude made.	Moon's age.	Winds.	Rain or Dew.	Appearances of the Atmosphere.	REMARKS, AND STATE OF THE SICK LIST.
1773 Maii 9	8 12 8	81 81 81	17° 28″ Beata		18	NE EbN *		c. cl.	The remittent returned 18th, ult. and 1 fcurvy added to the lift; 7 in it.
10	8 12 8	81 81 81	17° 45″	from Antavelle 01° 36″ W	19	NE EbN *		cl.	One fcurvy, and 1 contufion added to the lift; 9 in it. Thefe little iflands are clofe to Hifpaniola. I mean Beata, and Antavelle.
11	8 12 8	81 81 81	17° 00″	from Navaffa 00° 28″ W	20	NE EbN *		cl. c.	An old remittent fever added to the lift, with fcorbutick fymptoms; 10 in it. The afthma is highly fcorbutick.
12	8 12 8	82 84 83	Jamaica		21	Sb ***		c.	Sent the afthma, and the fcurvy of the 9th, to the hofpital; 8 in the lift. Anchored at Port Royal a. m. Sir George Rodney commands here ftill; but few of His Majefty's fhips in the harbour.
13	8 12 8	82 83 83			22	Sb & lb		cl. c.	Sent one fcurvy to the hofpital, who was not in the lift, 1 diarrhœa, and 3 fcurvies added to the lift; 12 in it. Frefh beef being allowed to the fhip but once a week, I folicited the Captain to apply to the Admiral for frefh meat for our men every meat day, as many of them were fcorbutick, but the Admiral would not grant it.
14	8 12 4 8	81 83 84 82			23	Sb & lb		c. cl.	Sent 10 fcorbuticks to the hofpital for the benefit of frefh diet, 1 of them was not in the lift, 2 contufions, 1 is the old opthalmia, he hurt his eye again, added to the lift; 5 in it. The water we get on board is brackifh, though there is as good water to be got as can be wifhed for.
15	8 12 4 8	82 83 81 83			24	Sb & lb		c. cl.	The old fcorbutick rheumatifm returned to duty, and the diarrhœa of the 13th well; 3 in the lift.
16	8 12 8	82 84 82			25	Sb & lb		c. cl.	One druken complaint added to the lift; 4 in it. Our men continually drunk with new rum.
17	8 12 8	82 84 82			26	Sb & lb		c. cl.	The contufion of the 10th, well; 2 accidents from drunkennefs, 1 fluxed complaint, and 1 ficknefs at ftomach added to the lift; 7 in it.
18	8 12 8	81 81 81			27	Sb & lb		c.	The ulcer of the 29th ult. and yefterday's diarrhœa well, 1 flux added to the lift; 6 in it.
19	8 12 8	80 81 81			28	Sb & lb		c.	The ficknefs at ftomach of the 17th, well, 5 in the lift.—Though the drunken complaint of the 16th is not in it, yefterday's flux is a bad dyfentery—a marine.

Year, Months, and Days.	Hours.	Thermometer.	Latitude or different parts.	Longitude made.	Moon's age.	Winds.	Rain or Dew.	Appearances of the Atmosphere.	REMARKS, AND STATE OF THE SICK LIST.
1773 Maii 20	8 12 8	81 82 82			29	Sb & lb		c.	Two fluxed, and 2 feverish complaints added to the lift; 9 in it.
21	8 12 8	82 82 83			m. p.m	Sb & lb		c.	One of the accidents of the 17th, well; and 1 flux added to the lift; 9 in it. 2 of yesterda fluxes io a dysentery.
22	8 12 8	81 84 82			1	Sb & lb		c.	The dysentery of the 18th, and 1 of the fevers of of the 20th, sent to the hospital. The contused eye of the 14th, the diarrhœa of the 20th, and 1 of the feverish complaints of the 20th, well; 4 in the lift.
23	8 12 8	81 82 82			2	Sb & lb		c.	No alteration in the lift.
24	8 12 8	81 81 81			3	Sb & lb		c.	The flux of the 21ft, is well; 3 fluxes, and 1 sickness at stomach, added to the lift; 8 in it. Besides some slight complaints.
25	8 12 8	81 81 81			4	Sb & lb		c.	The other accident of the 17th, the dysentery of the 20th, and 1 of yesterday's fluxed complaints well; 2 fevers, 1 of them was returned well of a diarrhœa the 15th, and 2 fluxes added to the lift; 9 in it.
26	8 12 8	81 78 78			5	V *	. . .	cl.	One same complaint added to the lift; 10 in it. A dysentery died at the hospital, and it has attacked the scorbutick men we sent there. The fluxes on board are dysenteries.
27	8 12 8	80 80 80			6	V *	. .	cl.	Sent 7 dysenteries, 1 was a slight complaint 24th, and 1 fever, to the hospital; Yesterday's complaint well, and 1 of the fevers of the 25th slight, 3 dysenteries, and 2 fever added to the lift; 5 in it.
28	8 12 8	80 80 80			7	V *	. .	cl.	Five dysenteries added to the lift; sent 7 and yesterday's fever to the hospital. And 1 contusion complained; 3 in the lift.
29	8 12 8	80 80 80			8	V *	.	cl.	The slight fever of the 25th well; and yesterday's contusion, 1 dysentery, and 1 with feverish symptoms added to the lift; 3 in it.
30	8 12 8	80 81 83			9	V *		c.	Yesterday's feverish complaint well, 3 with feverish symptoms, and 1 dysentery added to the lift; 6 in it.
31	8 12 8	81 81 83			10	Sb & lb		c.	Three with feverish symptoms, and 1 dysentery added to the lift; 10 in it. Eight returned from the hospital very weak.

Year, Months, and Days.	Hours.	Thermometer.	Latitude or different Parts.	Longitude made.	Moon's age.	Winds.	Rain or Dew.	Appearances of the Atmoſphere.	REMARKS, AND STATE OF THE SICK LIST.
1773 Junii 1 Die Martis	8 12 8	81 82 83	Jamaica		11	Sb & lb		c.	One of the feveriſh complaints of the 30th ult. well; 1 diarrhœa, and 1 rheumatiſm, who came from the hoſpital laſt night, added to the liſt; 11 in it. 5 Dyſenteries, 5 ſlight fevers, and 1 rheumatiſm.
2	8 12 8	81 82 83			12	Sb & lb		c.	One of the feveriſh complaints of the 31ſt ult. and yeſterday's diarrhœa, well; and ſent three fevers and 1 dyſentery to the hoſpital, 1 dyſentery added to the liſt; 6 in it.
3	8 12 8	81 82 82			13	Sb & lb		c.	One of the feveriſh complaints of the 30th, well 1 ſore throat, and 1 lame complaint added to the liſt; 7 in it,
4	8 12 8	81 82 82			p. p. m	Sb & lb		c.	The dyſenteries of the 29th and 30th ult. and of thn 1ſt, well; 2 dyſenteries, 1 old cough, and 1 ſlight complaint added to the liſt; 8 in it.
5	8 12 8	81 85 82			15	Sb & lb		c.	The dyſentery of the 31ſt, well; 2 dyſenteries and 1 with feveriſh ſymptoms added to the liſt 10 in it. The aſthma died of the dyſentery a the hoſpital.
6	8 12 8	82 85 83			16	Sb & lb		c. cl.	The ſlight complaint of the 4th, and yeſterday e feveriſh complaint, well; 1 of the dyſenteries of the 4th, ſent to the hoſpital, 1 flux, and 1 with feveriſh ſymptoms added to the liſt; 9 in it.
7	8 12 8	82 85 83			17	Sb & lb		cl.	The old cough well; 8 in the liſt.
8	8 12 8	82 85 84			18	Sb & lb		cl. c.	The complaints of the 3d, the dyſenteries of the 5th, and the feveriſh complaint of the 6th, well; 3 with feveriſh ſymptoms added to the liſt; 6 in it. Two ſcurvies, and 2 dyſenteries returned well from the hoſpital.
9	8 12 8	79 82 81			19	Sb & lb		cl. c.	One rheumatiſm (newly entered on board) added to the liſt; 7 in it.
10	8 12 8	80 82 82			20	Sb & lb		cl. c.	One with feveriſh ſymptoms added to the liſt; in it.
11	8 12 8	80 83 82			21	Sb & lb		cl. c.	The complaints of the 8th, the rheumatiſm of the 9th, and yeſterday's complaint, well; 1 dyſentery added to the liſt; 4 in it.
12	8 12 8	82 84 83			22	Sb & lb		cl	Two dyſenteries added to the liſt; 6 in it.

Year, Months, and Days.	Hours.	Thermometer	Latitude or different parts.	Longitude made.	Moon's Age	Winds.	Rain and Dew.	Appearances of the Atmosphere.	REMARKS, AND STATE OF THE SICK LIST.
1773 Junii 13	8 12 8	81 83 82	Jamaica		23	Sb & lb		cl.	The other dysentery of the 4th, and yesterday's, both sent to the hospital; 1 dysentery, 1 lame complaint, 1 intermitting headach, and 1 muscular pain of the side, added to the list; 8 in it.
14	8 12 8	81 83 82			24	Sb & lb		cl. c.	One dysentery, and 1 fever, who were both at the hospital, relapsed; 10 in the list.
15	8 12 8	81 83 82			25	Sb & lb		cl. c.	The flux of the 6th, well; 9 in the list. The muscular pain of the 13th, is a dysentery now. His Majesty's ship Princess Amelia, sailed for England.
16	8 12 8	81 83 82			26	Sb & lb		c. cl.	One dysentery added to the list; 10 in it. The Admiral sailed in His Majesty's ship Portland, on a cruize.
17	8 12 8	82 83 82			27	Sb & lb		cl.	The dysentery, and the lame complaint of the 13th, well; 8 in the list.
18	8 12 8	82 85 83			28	Sb & lb		cl. c.	The intermitting headach of the 18th, well; 2 dysenteries, and a hæmorrhage added to the list. His Majesty's ship Guadaloupe came in The thermometer ashore 91 at noon.
19	8 12 8	84 85 83			29	Sb & lb		cl. c.	One dysentery who returned as well from the hospital, relapsed; 11 in the list. P. m. the men were brought off from the hospital, 1 died last night of the dysentery, and 1 some day ago Very hot.
20	8 12 8	82 84 83			m. a. m.	Sb & lb		cl. c.	Ten dysenteries of them who returned yesterday from the hospital, and 1 scurvy who was there, 1 with feverish symptoms, 1 strain, and 1 scorbutick swelling, added to the list; 24 in it.
21	8 12 8	83 83 81			2	Sb & lb		cl. c.	Yesterday's hospital scurvy does duty, 1 contusion added to the list; 24 in it. The hospital dysenteries are very weak. Sailed at 6 a. m. fell in with His Majesty's ships, Portland, Princess Amelia, and Seaford; and joined company with them, by the admiral's order.
22	8 12 8	82 82 82	Blue fields		3	Sb & lb		cl. h.	The dysentery of the 16th, and the strain of the 20th, well; 4 dysenteries, and 1 with feverish symptoms added to the list; 27 in it. The hospital fluxes all rather better, of 18 fluxes 11 are marines. Anchored at noon.
23	8 12 8	82 85 82			4	V	. . . p. m	h. cl. t. l.	The dysentery who was the muscular pain of the 13th, the old hospital fever of the 14th, 1 dysentery of the 18th, and the feverish complaint of the 20th, well; 23 in the list. The weak fluxes complain more to-night.

Year, Months, and Days.	Hours.	Thermometer.	Latitude or different parts.	Longitude made.	Moon's age.	Winds.	Rain or Dew.	Appearances of the Atmosphere.	REMARKS, AND STATE OF THE SICK LIST.
1773 Junii 24	8 12 8	82 85 83			5	V	. . . p.	h. cl.	One of the hospital, took ill the 25th ult. and 1 of the 22d dysenteries, well; 1 dysentery added to the list; 22 in it. We lie under very high mountains, from whence there is either a constant fog, or rain, and receive none of the benefit of the sea breeze, but have frequent disagreeable puffs of wind off the mountains. The water is remarkably fine ashore; and limes very plenty.
25	8 12 8	83 85 83			6	V a. m. p. m. Sb	. . .	h. cl.	The feverish complaint of the 22d well; and 1 dy- added to the list; 22 in it. All the fluxes, especially the hospital ones, much weaker and worse. P. m. all the squadron sailed.
26	8 12 8	82 84 83			7	a. m. EbN p. m. NbW **		h. cl.	The flux of the 24th, well; 21 in the list. A. m. stood off and on towards the land; p. m. we and the Princess Amelia, parted company with the Portland and Seaford,
27	8 12 8	83 84 83	19° 02″	from the West End Jamaica 02°05″ W	8	ENE **		cl. c.	Two dysenteries, 1 of them was the hospital fever of the 20th ult. the other is of the 22d instant, recovered; 19 in the list. The Princess Amelia in company.
28	8 12 8	84 84 83	20° 02″	03°58″ W	9	NE ENE **		h. cl.	One of the hospital fluxes of the 28th ult. died, and two of them, 1 took ill the 27th ult. and the other 13th inst. well; the hospital flux who relapsed on the 14th, is a vomica, as well as being dysenterick; 16 in the list.
29	8 12 8	84 83 82	21° 19″	04°59″ W	10	V *		h. cl.	One hospital flux, took ill the 28th ult. recovered, 1 feverish complaint, and 1 rheumatism added the list; 17 in it.
30	8 12 8	84 83 82	21° 42″	from the West End of the Isle of Pines 00° 34″ W	11	ENE lb. *		cl.	Two fluxes, 1 an hospital one, took ill the 4th, and the other the 22d. and yesterday's feverish complaint, well, 1 flux added to the list; 14 in it. The scorbutick swelling of the 20th, has got a flux from attending the sick.
Julii 1 Die Jovis	8 12 4 8	82 82 83 82	21° 43″	Cape Orientis	12	f EbN t NNW *		cl. c.	Four fluxes added to the list; 18 in it. 14 Fluxes, 1 fever, 1 rheumatism, 1 contusion, and 1 vomica. Sailing along Cuba.
2	8 2 3 8	83 84 85 111S 85	22° 06″		13	*		h. c.	One of the fluxes took ill the 11th ult. died, both of them who died, marines; 1 flux added to the list; 18 in it. P. m. the sun's rays were very hot. The thermometer rose therein in a few minutes, 26 degrees.
3	8 12 8	85 84 83	22° 39″		14	ENE *		c.	One flux, who was an attendant of the sick, added to the list; 19 in it. The flux who was took ill the 19th of May, is recovered; but has a large ulcer.

Year, Months, and Days.	Hours.	Thermometer.	Latitude or different parts.	Longitude made.	Moon's age.	Winds.	Rain or Dew.	Appearances of the Atmosphere.	REMARKS, AND STATE OF THE SICK LIST.
1773 Julii 4	8 12 8	85 85 85	23° 06″	from Cap St. Anthony 00° 12″ W	p. a. m.	V *		c.	One hofpital flux, took ill the 27th May, 1 flux of the 21ft, and the rheumatifm of the 29th ult. well; 1 old hofpital flux, and the old fcorbutick rheumatifm relapfed; 18 in the lift.
5	8 12 8	84 85 84	23° 00″	00° 19″ E	16	V *		p. m. cl.	The dyfentery of the 25th ult. well; 1 flux, and 1 hypochondria, added to the lift; 19 in it. Very hot.
6	8 12 8	84 85 84	22° 42″	00° 49″ E	17	V *		cl. c.	Yefterday's hypochondria well; 18 in the lift.
7	8 12 8	83 82 81	23° 00″ Off Cuba		18	f SSE t ENE *	.	cl. c.	No alteration in the fick lift. Standing off and on towards Cuba.
8	8 12 8	83 83 83	23° 01″		19	f NNE t ESE *		c.	One of the fluxes of the 1ft, added to the lift, is well; and an old fcorbutick complaint added to the lift; 18 in it.
9	8 12 8	83 84 83	23° 02″		20	f NNE t ESE **		c.	The flux of the 30th ult. 2 of the 1ft, and the relapfed hofpital one of the 4th well; 14 in the lift.
10	8 12 8	83 83 82	23° 21″ Havannah		21	**		p. m. cl.	No alteration in the lift.
11	8 12 8	82 83 82	23° 30″		22	f SbE t EbN **	. .	cl.	One hofpital fever took ill 31ft May, 1 hofpital flux, relapfed the 19th ult. the flux of the 2d, and the fcorbutick complaint of the 8th, well; 2 fluxes (relapfed ones) added to the lift; 12 in it.
12	8 12 8	83 83 82	24° 16″	from Matanfa 00° 32″ E	23	E *		h.	The fcorbutick fwelling of the 20th ult. recovered of his flux, and the yefterday's well flux of the 2d. relapfed; 12 in the lift.
13	8 12 5 8	83 83 86 84	25° 03″	00° 42″ E	24	E *		h. cl.	One marine hofpital flux, took ill the 12th ult. died; 2 fluxes, 1 of the 18th, and the other of the 22d ult. recovered; 9 in the lift.
14	8 12 8	83 83 83	25° 44″	00° 53″ E	25	E ***	.	cl.	One contufion added to the lift; 10 in it. Squally at times.
15	8 12 8	83 83 83	27° 18″	01° 02″ E	26	V *		c.	Yefterday's contufion well; 9 in the lift. Lost fight of the Princefs Amelia; 3 men came on board from a merchant fhip, with very large foul ulcers to be dreffed. I fpared them fome bark and dreffings.

Year, Months, and Days.	Hours.	Thermometer	Latitude or different parts.	Longitude made.	Moon's Age	Winds.	Rain and Dew.	Appearances of the Atmosphere.	REMARKS, AND STATE OF THE SICK LIST.
1773 Julii 16	8 12 4 8	83 82 84 83	29° 21″	01° 40″ E	27	f WbS t SWbS		cl. c.	The old scorbutick rheumatism, and the relapsed flux of the 12th, well; 1 flux, and 1 feverish complaint added to the list; 9 in it.
17	8 12 8	83 83 83	30° 31″	03° 18″ E	28	f WbS t SWbS		cl. h.	One flux added to the list; 10 in it. Very sultry.
18	8 12 8	82 81 80	31° 13″	05° 08″ E	29	*		cl. c.	The feverish complaint of the 16th, and yesterday's, well; 1 flux, and 1 feverish complaint added to the list; 10 in it.
19	8 12 8	80 79 80	30° 17″	06° 15″ E	m. p. m.	f NbE t NEbE *		cl.	One flux of the 1st, 1 of the 5th, 1 of the 11th, and yesterday's complaints, well; 1 suppressed perspiration added to the list; 6 in it.
20	8 12 8	80 81 80	30° 18″	06° 25″ E	1	ESE *		c.	One complaint with eruptions added to the list; in it.
21	8 12 8	81 82 82	31° 21″	06° 59″ E	2	f SW t W *		cl.	The flux of the 11th, returned 19th, relapsed from irregularities, and 1 flux added to the list; 9 in it. The vomica recovers a pace.
22	8 12 8	81 81 79	32° 27″	08° 28″ E	3	f SW t NW ***	. . .	cl. t. l.	The complaint of the 20th, well; 8 in the list
23	8 12 8	80 81 80	32° 47″	08° 54″ E	4	a. m. * p. m. S	.	cl.	The flux of the 16th, and the complaint of the 19th, well; 6 in the list. The valetudinarian fluxes are much affected with the change of weather.
24	8 12 8	81 80 80	34° 12″ R	10° 40″ E	5	S **	. .	cl.	The vomica again seized with his flux, and is much worse. No alteration in the list.
25	8 12 8	79 78 78	35° 50″ R	14° 05″ E	6	f S t WSW *	. .	cl.	No alteration in the list.
26	8 12 8	79 79 78	37° 27″	17° 21″ E	7	f SSW t SSE **		cl. c.	Six in the list. Disagreeable weather.
27	8 12 8	79 79 78	38° 28″	18° 04″ E	8	SSW t SSE **		cl. c.	No alteration in the list.
28	8 12 8	79 80 79	40° 06″	19° 41″ E	9	V a. m. *** p. m. S		cl.	The list continues the same.

Year, Months, and Days.	Hours.	Thermometer.	Latitude of different Parts.	Longitude made.	Moon's age.	Winds.	Rain or Dew.	Appearances of the Atmosphere.	REMARKS, AND STATE OF THE SICK LIST.
1773 Julii 29	8 12 4 8	78 78 80 78	40° 36″	22° 18″ E	10	p. m. SbW **	.	cl.	The vomica died of his flux in the night. The flux of the 3d, the other one of the 11th, and the relapsed one of the 21st, well; 2 in the list.
30	8 12 8	79 79 78	41° 20″	25° 28″ E	11	SbW***	.	cl. c.	No alteration in the list. The old scorbutick rheumatism, has been ailing again since the rainy weather began.
31	8 12 8	78 78 76	42° 02″	28° 43″ E	12	S *		c.	No alteration in the list. The 2 in it, are the flux of the 21st ult. and the ulcer'd man, who was the flux added May 28th.
Aug. 1 Die Sabbati	8 12 8	77 79 78	42° 33″	31° 09″ E	13	V p. m. ***	. .	cl. t. l.	One bad flux, a marine took ill yesterday, 1 with sore eyes, and 1 headach, added to the list; 5 in it.
2	8 12 8	74 73 72	43° 16″	31° 29″ E	p. p. m.	E **		cl. h.	No alteration in the list. A cold disagreeable day.
3	8 12 4 8	72 72 74 73	43° 39″	31° 29″ E	15	ESE SE **		cl. h.	Five in the list.
4	8 12 8	72 72 70	44° 56″	32° 39″ E	16	f SEbS t ESE ***	. . . .	h. cl.	The list continues the same.
5	8 12 8	68 70 69	45° 58″	33° 02″ E	17	f EbN t SEbE	.	cl. h.	The relapsed hospital flux, returned well, the 11th ult. added again to the list; 6 in it. Very cold.
6	8 12 8	67 68 68	46° 07″	35° 12″ E	18	f EbN t N	. .	h. cl.	One old hospital flux relapsed; 7 in the list.
7	8 12 8	68 67 67	45° 52″	35° 12″ E	19	V *		cl.	The headach of the 1st, well; 6 in the list.
8	8 12 8	66 66 66	45° 35″	37° 04″ E	20	N **	.	cl.	The bad dysentery of the 1st, died, a bad fever attended it, 2 fluxes, 1 of them an old hospital one, and was took ill a fortnight ago though he did not complain, is now exceedingly ill, relapsed, and 1 relapsed rheumatism added to the list; 8 in it.
9	8 12 8	66 65 68	45° 52″	39° 20″ E	21	f NW t SbW **	.	cl. h.	The sore eyes of the 1st, well; 7 in the list.

Year, Months, and Days	Hours.	Thermometer.	Latitude or different parts.	Longitude made.	Moon's age.	Winds.	Rain or Dew.	Appearances of the Atmosphere.	REMARKS, AND STATE OF THE SICK LIST.
1773 Aug. 10	8 12 8	70 69 69	46° 25″	43° 27″ E	22	f SbW tWbN***	.	h. cl.	An old flux relapsed; 8 in the list.
11	8 12 8	65 65 64	46° 35″	46° 47″ E	23	f NbE t NW***	.	h. cl.	An old flux relapsed; 9 in the list.
12	8 12 8	64 63 65	46° 36″	49° 32″ E	24	NW **		cl.	The rheumatism of the 8th, well; 8 in the list.
13	8 12 8	65 66 66	47° 12″	52° 22″ E	25	f W t SWbW **	.	cl.	One flux added to the list; 9 in it.
14	8 12 8	65 66 66	48° 12″	56° 40″ E	26	f WSW t NW ***	.	cl. c.	The old relapsed hospital flux, added the 8th, died, and the flux added the 6th, well; 7 in the list.
15	8 12 8	63 64 64	48° 42″	59° 20″ E	27	f WbS t ENE *	.	h. cl.	No alteration in the list.
16	8 12 8	63 63 63	49° 04″	60° 46″ E	28	f N t NW***	.	cl. h.	Seven in the list. Very cold.
17	8 12 8	63 65 63	49° 11″	64° 16″ E	29	V *	. .	cl. h.	One contusion added to the list; 8 in it.
18	8 12 8	64 63 63	49° 15″	65° 23″ E	m. a. m.	f E t NNW ***	.	c. h.	One with a dimness of sight added to the list; 9 in it.
19	8 12 8	63 63 63	49° 31″ p. m. Scilly	68° 14″ E	2	NNW	.	cl. h.	One cough, an old man, added to the list; 10 in it.
20	8 12 8	63 63 63	49° 55″		3	a. m. * p. m. E		c. cl.	One of the relapsed fluxes of the 8th, well; and an old relapsed hospital flux added to the list; 10 in it. Yesterday's complaint, has had a colliquative flux on him this month past, but did not complain.
21	8 12 8	63 64 63	49° 00″		4	V *		cl. c.	The ulcer'd complaint, who was a flux, and the flux of the 13th, well; 2 contusions, and the old scorbutick swelling of the 20th June, who was fluxed too, become more scorbutick and added to the list; 11 in it.
22	8 12 8	65 67 70	Off the land		5	V *	❖	c.	The complaint with a dimness of sight, well; 1 flux, and 1 abscess added to the list; 12 in it.

Year, Months, and Days.	Hours.	Thermometer.	Latitude or different parts.	Longitude made.	Moon's age.	Winds.	Rain or Dew.	Appearances of the Atmosphere.	REMARKS, AND STATE OF THE SICK LIST.
1773 Aug. 23	8 12 8	67 68 70	50° 25″		6	V *	❖	c. h.	The complaint of the 19th, and 1 of the contusions of the 21st, well; 1 old contusion added to the list with a flux; 11 in it.
24	8 12	66 67	1 p. m Cowes		7	W *	❖	c. h.	No alteration in the list. Last night we lay at an anchor off the Needles, and this morning sailed, and anchor'd in Cowes Road at 1 p. m. To be sent to the hospital, 5 valetudinarian fluxes, and 2 old rheumatick complaints. Sick on board, 3 slight fluxes, 1 took ill the 9th, 1 the 22d, and the other 23d, 1 contusion of the 17th, 1 of the 21st, 1 scurvy of the 21st, the abscess of the 22d, none of them bad, and the old scorbutick rheumatism.

END OF THE SECOND VOYAGE.

CHAPTER III.

The Diary of the Weather and State of the Sick List, between the 21ſt of November 1773, and the 1ſt of September 1774.

Year, Months, and Days.	Hours.	Thermometer	Latitude or different parts.	Longitude made.	Moon's Age	Winds.	Rain and Dew.	Appearances of the Atmosphere.	REMARKS, AND STATE OF THE SICK LIST.
1773 Nov. 21 Die Sabbati	8 12 8	58 f 58 f 60 f	49° 59″		8	f NE t NbE **		cl.	Sailed laft evening with His Majefty's Sloop Weafel from Cowes; 7 in the lift—2 foul ulcers, 1 feverifh complaint, 1 ftrain, 1 rheumatifm, 1 piles, and 1 weak from a fever.
22	8 12 8	54 f 54 f 58 f	Off Scilly		9	f SWbS t N ***	. .	cl.	The feverifh complaint, well; 6 in the lift, M. The Weafel put about and ftood from us. Very cold and difagreeable.
23	8 12 8	54 f 54 f 61 f	48° 01″	from Scilly 02° 18″ W	10	f SW t NW ***	. .	cl.	No alteration in the lift.
24	8 12 8	55 f 57 f 64 f	46° 39″	02° 35″ W	11	f NNW t ENE **		cl. c.	One contufion, and 1 inflammation added to the lift; 8 in it; but fome of them do duty.
25	8 12 8	55 f 57 f 65 f	45° 16″	03° 55″ W	12	f NNW t ENE **		cl. c.	One contufion added to the lift; 9 in it. Agreeable weather.
26	8 12 8	57 60 f 67 f	43° 36″	06° 01″ W	13	f ENE t ESE **		cl: c.	The piles of the 21, well; 8 in the lift.
27	8 12 8	61 64 f 70 f	40° 50″	07° 10″ W	14	f SE t SSE **		cl. c.	The weak complaint of the 21ft, and the contufion of the 24th, well; the returned feverifh complaint of the 22d, relapfed; 7 in the lift.
28	8 12 8	64 70 f 70 f	39° 02″	08° 09″ W	p. p. m·	f SSE t SE **		cl. c.	The rheumatifm, and yefterday's complaint, well· 5 in the lift. The contufion of the 25th is a remitting fever.
29	8 12 8	66 71 f 71 f	37° 33″	08° 57″ W	16	f SSE t SE **		cl. c.	One inflammation added to the lift; 6 in it.
30	8 12 8	68 71 f 71 f	36° 02″	09° 40″ W	17	f SE t SbE **		cl. c.	No alteration in the lift. 3 Ulcers, 2 inflammations, and 1 fcorbutick complaint, who was the ftrain of the 21ft.
Dec. 1 Die Mercurii	8 12 8	67 67 67	34° 31″	09° 58″ W	18	SEbE **		cl. c.	One ulcer added to the lift; 7 in it.
2	8 12 8	67 66 68	32° 24″	10° 11″ W	19	f ESE t SE **		cl. c.	No alteration in the lift.
3	8 12 8	68 68 68	30° 51″	10° 32″ W	20	f ESE t SE **		cl. c.	Seven in the lift.

Year, Months, and Days.	Hours.	Thermometer.	Latitude or different Parts.	Longitude made.	Moon's age.	Winds.	Rain or Dew.	Appearances of the Atmosphere.	REMARKS, AND STATE OF THE SICK LIST.
1773 Dec. 4	8 12 8	68 68 70	28° 28″ St. Cruze Teneriffe		21	f ESE t SE **		cl. c.	The inflammation of the 24th, and the contufion of the 25th, fince the remitting fever, well; 1 feverifh, and 1 gravelifh complaints added to the lift; 7 in it.
5	8 12 8	69 70 69			22	Sb & lb		c. cl.	No alteration in the lift. Some of the men, as is ufual, drunk from getting wine off from St. Cruze. No ftock to be got, and fcarce any vegetables. We always lye above a mile from the wharf.
6	8 12 8	68 67 67			23	Sb & lb		c. cl.	Seven in rhe lift.
7	8 12 8	69 68 67			24	Sb & lb		cl.	The feverifh complaint of the 4th, well; 6 in the lift.
8	8 12 8	68 70 67			25	Sb & lb		cl. c.	One rheumatifm who was the feverifh complaint of the 21ft, and 1 purging complaint, added to the lift; 8 in it.
9	8 12 8	68 69 69			26	Sb & lb		cl. c.	No alteration in the lift.
10	8 12 8	70 70 69			27	Sb & lb		cl. c.	The purging complaint of the 8th, well; 7 in the lift.
11	8 12 8	70 70 71			28	Sb & lb		cl. c.	No alteration in the lift. A. m. the Weafel came in. After fhe put about on the 22d ult. they met with a gale of wind and went back to England.
12	8 12 8	67 70 73 f			29	Sb & lb		cl. c.	One feverifh complaint added to the lift; 8 in it.
13	8 12 8	70 71 72 f			m. p. m.	Sb & lb		cl. c.	The rheumatifm of the 8th, well; 1 fwelled face added to the lift; 8 in it. P. m. His Majefty's fhips Salifbury, and Sea Horfe, went paft.
14	8 12 8	70 70 72 f			1	Sb & lb		cl. c.	The gravelifh complaint of the 4th, well; 7 in the lift.
15	8 12 8	70 70 75 f			2	Sb & lb		c. cl.	The fwelled face of the 13th, well; 1 feverifh complaint, and 1 fwelled face, added to the lift; 8 in it. The complaint of the 12th, is a remittent fever.
16	8 12 8	70 71 70			3	Sb & lb		c. cl.	Yefterday's feverifh complaint, well; 1 complaint with eruptions, and 1 fwelled face added to the lift. Thefe fwelled faces, are attended with a fever, fhall therefore call them a catarrhous fever.

Year, Months, and Days.	Hours.	Thermometer.	Latitude or different parts.	Longitude made.	Moon's age.	Winds.	Rain or Dew.	Appearances of the Atmosphere.	REMARKS, AND STATE OF THE SICK LIST.
1773									ver. The water and wine which we got on board were as good as ufual; 9 in the lift. Sailed with the Weafel at 5 p. m.
Dec. 17	8 12 8	71 71 72	28° 04″		4	V *		c. cl.	One catarrhous fever added to the lift; 10 in it.
18	8 12 8	71 71 71	26° 54″	from St. Cruze 00° 19″ E	5	W *		c. cl.	The feverifh complaint of the 4th, and the catarrhous fever of the 15th, well; 1 catarrhous fever added to the lift; 9 in it.
19	8 12 8	70 70 70	25° 23″ Coaft of Barbary	01° 00″ E	6	W WSW *		c. cl.	The complaint with eruptions of the 16th, well; 1 abfcefs added to the lift; 9 in it.
20	8 12 8	69 69 69	25° 02″	01° 02″ E	7	f W t SW **	.	cl.	The remitting fever of the 12, well; 1 catarrhous fever, and 1 contufion added to the lift; 10 in it.
21	8 12 8	69 69 69	24° 50″	00° 47″ E	8	f N t NW *	.	cl. h.	No alteration in the lift. The fea has a very difagreeable fmell. Anchor'd from 9 a. m. to 1 p. m.
22	8 12 8	70 68 68	24° 32″	00° 37″ E	9	f NW t NE *	.	c.	Ten in the lift.
23	8 12 8	66 65 65	23° 36″	00° 47″ W	10	ENE **		c.	One catarrhous fever of the 17th, 1 of the 18th, and the abfcefs of the 19th, well; 7 in the lift.
24	8 12 8	65 65 67	20 47″ Cape Blancho		11	ENE **		c.	The contufion of the 20th, well; and the remitting fever returned to duty the 20th, is relapfed. M. anchor'd off Cape Blancho, very cold.
25	8 12 8	67 69 70			12	f NNE t ENE **	✤	c.	One feverifh complaint added to the lift; 8 in it. The fhore feems to be quite a defert. Our boats went a fifhing laft night, and caught with the feene a great many very large fifh, both flat and round; fome of the latter weighed 84lb. each, and were exceedingly fat. Their proper names I know not. We lye about 2 miles from the fhore.
26	8 12 8	68 68 67	20° 44″		13	f NNE t ENE *	✤	c.	The catarrhous fever of the 20th, is become a very bad cough; 8 in the lift. Sailed at 9 a. m. with the Weafel.
27	8 12 8	63 67 69	19° 14″	from Cape Blancho 00° 08″ E	14	f NNE t ENE *	✤	c.	The Catarrhous fever of the 16th; and the feverifh complaint of the 25th, well; 6 in the lift. The land is very low, which we are failing paft.

Year, Months, and Days.	Hours.	Thermometer.	Latitude or different parts.	Longitude made.	Moon's age.	Winds.	Rain or Dew.	Appearances of the Atmosphere.	REMARKS, AND STATE OF THE SICK LIST.
1773 Dec. 28	8 12 8	68 67 68	18° 27″	01° 05″ E	15	f NNE t ENE *	✥	c.	One catarrhous fever added to the lift; 7 in it. 6 p. m. anchor'd about 5 or 6 miles from the fhore.
29	8 12 8	68 67 70	17° 58″	01° 26″ E	p. a. m.	f NNE t ENE *	✥	h.	Two ulcers, 1 of the 21ft ult. and 1 of the 1ft, well; 2 contufions added to the lift; 7 in it. A great many large groupers and fnappers caught along fide of the fhip with bait. Sailed at 9 a. m. and anchor'd at 2 p. m. with the Weafel.
30	8 12 8	69 70 70	17° 58″	01° 26″ E	17	f NNE t ENE *	✥	h.	No alteration in the lift. At 1 p. m. failed and anchored again at 6 p. m. By anchoring fo often we endeavoured to find out with the boats, a place called Portendick; but to no purpofe.
31	8 12 8	70 69 69	17° 30″	01° 16″ E	18	f NNE t ENE *	✥	h.	The relapfed fever of the 24th, well; and 1 feverifh complaint, added to the lift; 7 in it. Two contufions, 1 fcurvy, 1 very bad cough, 1 remitting fever, 1 catarrhous fever, and 1 ulcer. Sailed at 9 a. m.
1774 Jan. 1 Die Saturni	8 12 8	69 69 69	16° 23″ Senegal road	01° 17″ E	19	f NNE t ENE **	✥	h.	No alteration in the lift. 5 P. m. anchored in the road off Senegal bar, about 5 miles from the fhore; 5 merchant fhips lying here, to get over the bar; but it has been fo rough of late, that 1 of them has been waiting thefe fix weeks paft, and could not even fend a boat over.
2	8 12 4 8	68 70 71 70	15° 53″		20	f NNW t ENE **	✥	h.	One inflammation added to the lift; 8 in it. A good deal of fwell here. The Weafel in company with us.
3	8 12 4 8	69 70 72 71			21	f NNW t ENE **	✥	h.	No alteration in the lift.
4	8 12 8	70 71 71			22	f NNW t ENE **	✥	h.	Eight in the lift. No boat can pafs the bar yet. A very thick haze or fog, with a fwell.
5	8 12 8	71 71 72			23	f NNW t ENE	✥	h.	The catarrhous fever of the 28th, well; and 1 of the contufions, the right elbow, of the 29th ult. returned to duty though not quite well; 1 catarrhous complaint, 1 with gripes, and 1 lame complaint, added to the lift; 9 in it. Difagreeable cold foggy weather. Severe wandering *mufcular* pains are very general on board.
6	8 12 8	72 71 71			24	f NNW t ENE **	✥	cl. h.	No alteration in the lift. Nor can a boat get over the bar.
7	8 12 8	71 73 74			25	f NNW t ENE	✥	cl. h.	The complaint of the 31ft, well; the recovered catarrhous complaints of the 5th, relapfed, and 2 more complained, 1 of them flight and not added to the lift; 10 in it.

U

Year, Months, and Days.	Hours.	Thermome-ter.	Latitude or different Parts.	Longitude made.	Moon's age.	Winds.	Rain or Dew.	Appearances of the At-mosphere.	REMARKS, AND STATE OF THE SICK LIST.
1774 Jan. 8	8 12 4 8	72 74 76 74	Senegal road		26	f NNW t ENE **	❖	h.	The griped complaint of the 5th, well; 9 in the lift. The bad cough is now become a bad fever.
9	8 12 8	72 73 72			27	f NNW t ENE **	❖	h.	One of the lame complaints is a venereal: 8 in the lift. A great fwell, and furf upon the bar yet.
10	8 12 8	72 72 72			28	f NNW t ENE ***	❖	h.	No alteration in the lift. A very thick fog.
11	8 12 8	72 72 71			29	f NNW t ENE ***	❖	h.	The inflammation of the 2d, well; 7 in the lift.
12	8 12 8	70 70 70			m. a. m.	f NNW t ENE ***	❖	h.	Two of the catarrhous complaints of the 7th, well; 5 in the lift.
13	8 12 8	70 70 71			2	f NNW t ENE *	❖	h. c.	The catarrhous complaint of the 5th, and the other of the 7th, well; 1 lame complaint, added to the lift; 4 in it.
14	8 12 4 8	70 70 72 74			3	f NNW t ENE *	❖	c.	One feverifh complaint, added to the lift; 5 in it. One of our boats, and one of the Weafel's gone over the bar.
15	8 12 8	71 71 75			4	Sb & lb	❖	c.	No alteration in the lift. The bad fever of the 8th, better. The fea and land breezes are more regular.
16	8 12 8	72 76 75			5	Sb & lb	❖	c. h.	The other contufion of the 29th ult. and the complaint of the 14th, well; 3 in the lift.
17	8 12 8	73 75 75			6	Sb & lb	❖	h.	No alteration in the lift.
18	8 12 8	73 75 75			7	Sb & lb *	❖	h. c.	One feverifh complaint with a tumour, added to the lift; 4 in it. A large fwell.
19	8 12 8	71 78 75			8	Sb & lb	❖	h. c.	One feverifh complaint, and 1 contufion added to the lift; 6 in it. The bad fever of the 8th remits now. The land wind remarkably hot.

Year, Months, and Days.	Hours.	Thermometer	Latitude or different parts.	Longitude made.	Moon's Age	Winds.	Rain and Dew.	Appearances of the Atmoſphere.	REMARKS, AND STATE OF THE SICK LIST.
1774 Jan. 20	8 12 4 8	71 76 79 77	Senegal Road		9	Sb & lb	❖	h. c.	No alteration in the liſt. The land wind has blown a great many different kinds of flies on board theſe two days.
21	8 12 8	72 73 76			10	Sb & lb	❖	h. c.	One feveriſh complaint added to the liſt; 7 in it. A ſhip arrived from Teneriffe, by which we are informed that a report prevailed there of our being caſt away on Cape Blancho, together with the Weaſel.
22	8 12 8	72 74 74			11	Sb & lb	❖	h. c.	The other ulcer of the 21ſt Nov. and yeſterday's complaint, well; 5 in the liſt. I conſulted Captain Collingwood about making a quarter caſk of wine, into a tincture of bark (ſee the poſtſcript) and got him to recommend the ſame method on board of the Weaſel.
23	8 12 8	72 72 73			12	Sb & lb	❖	h. c.	No alteration in the liſt. The bar unpaſſable yet.
24	8 12 8	72 73 72			13	Sb & lb	❖	h.	Five in the liſt.
25	8 12 8	71 71 71			14	Sb & lb	❖	h.	No alteration in the liſt.
26	8 12 8	71 72 72			15	Sb & lb	❖	h.	The complaints of the 19th, well; the boats returned p. m. Their crews were ſeized with ſevere gripings and a purging, while they waited on the beach for a ſmooth bar. There they made a ſort of tent, and lay ſome in it, and others in the boats, but not well covered from the dews; and they had only brackiſh water.
27	8 12 8	72 74 73			p. p. m.	Sb & lb	❖	h. c.	Three in the liſt. Captain Collingwood commiſſioned the Lord Dartmouth armed Schooner, and ſent on board of her a Captain, a Lieutenant, a ſurgeon, two midſhipmen, petty officers and men.
28	8 12 8	72 73 73			17	Sb & lb	❖	h. c.	The complaint of the 18th, well; and 1 with feveriſh ſymptoms added to the liſt; 3 in it. We got nothing from the ſhore of any kind.
29	8 12 8	72 73 73			18	Sb & lb	❖	c. h.	One feveriſh complaint added to the liſt; 4 in it. P. m got under way and anchored again.
30	8 12 4 8	72 72 74 73	15° 46″		19	N NbW**	❖	h. c.	Three added to the liſt with feveriſh complaints; 7 in it. Sailed at 9 a. m. with the Weaſel.

Year, Months, and Days.	Hours.	Thermometer.	Latitude or different parts.	Longitude made.	Moon's age.	Winds.	Rain or Dew.	Appearances of the Atmosphere.	REMARKS, AND STATE OF THE SICK LIST.
1774 Jan. 31	8 12 8	74 74 74	15° 34″	from Barbary Point 02° 10″ W	20	f NbW t NEbN ***		c.	The same complaint of the 13th, well; 6 in the list. 5 slight fevers, and 1 scurvy
Feb. 1 Die Martis	8 12 8	74 74 74	15° 11″	04° 58″ W	21	f NbW t NEbN **		c.	Two of the feverish complaints of the 30th, well 5 in the list
2	8 12 8	75 76 77	15° 15″ Mayo		22	f N t E		c.	The complaint of the 28th, well; 4 in the list. P. m. anchor'd at the isle of Mayo, with the Weasel.
3	8 12 4 8	75 77 79 77	15° 07″		23	f N t E		c.	No alteration in the list. Every thing in the fields ashore is burned up for want of rain; and every living creature as well as the people are almost starved, and they say that the drought has been general amongst the islands, and that there is a plague in some of them. We got a few bullocks on board, which are very lean indeed. They have very little live stock, and are in great want of provisions.
4	8 12 4 8	75 75 77 75			24	f N t E		c.	No alteration in the list.
5	8 12 8	74 75 77	St. Jago		25	p. m. V *		c.	The other slight fever of the 30th, well; 3 in the list. Sailed and anchored in Porto Prayo Bay, at 11 a. m. An English East India Packet lying here, that put in to refit after a violent storm of wind, thunder, and lightning, which we met with off the Cape Finister, and which, they inform us on board of her, did great damage at Madeira.
6	8 12 8	74 75 75			26	V *	.	cl.	No alteration in the list. No stock to be got, nor any kind of vegetables.
7	8 12 8	75 75 76			27	*	.	cl.	The feverish complaint of the 29th ult. well; 2 in the list. We caught a great many fish with the scene, and after supplying the Weasel and Packet there were a good many left, which were sent ashore to the Fort and received very thankfully by the governor. Sailed at 6 p. m. and left the Weasel.
8	8 12 8	75 75 76	14° 00″	from Porto Prayo 01° 01″ E	28	f E t NEbN **		cl.	The old bad cough, and fever, well; the scurvy in the list only.
9	8 12 8	70 75 75	12° 45″	02° 43″ E	29	NEbE **		h.	No alteration in the list.

Year, Months, and Days.	Hours.	Thermometer.	Latitude or different Parts.	Longitude made.	Moon's age.	Winds.	Rain or Dew.	Appearances of the Atmosphere.	REMARKS, AND STATE OF THE SICK LIST.
1774 Feb. 10	8 12 8	75 74 75	11° 26″	04° 29″ E	m. p. m.	f NEbE **		h.	One griped complaint added to the list; 2 in it.
11	8 12 4 8	75 76 77 76	10° 41″	from St. Jago 05° 22″ E	1	f NEbN t NW **		h. c.	Yesterday's complaint, well; 1 in the list.
12	8 12 8	76 78 77	10° 17″	06° 21″ E	2	V *		h. c.	One with eruptions, and 1 strain added to the list 3 in it.
13	8 12 4 8	78 79 80 79	10° 14″	06° 36″ E	3	a. m. — p.m.f NW t NbW *		h. c.	The 1 with eruptions does duty; and 1 diarrhœa added to the list; 3 in it. I made a quarter cask of wine into tincture of bark.
14	8 12 4 8	77 79 80 79	09° 21″	07° 26″ E	4	f NW t NbW **		h. c.	The strain of the 12th, well; 2 in the list.
15	8 12 8	79 78 79	08° 51″	08° 45″ E	5	f NW t NbW *	✣	h. c.	The diarrhœa of the 13th, well; 1 feverish complaint added to the list; 2 in it.
16	8 12 8	78 78 81	08° 29″		6	a. m. *** p. m. * NE	. . ✣	cl.	The complaint returned well the 7th again added to the list, with feverish symptoms; 3 in the list. A. m. anchored off Sierra Leon. P. m. Sailed and anchored in the river.
17	8 12 8	80 82 83	Sierra Leon		7	Sb & lb	✣	cl. h.	One diarrhœa added to the list; 4 in it. We lye as usual in Freeman's bay, very near the shore, 2 merchant ships in the bay; one of which has been very sickly, and buried 10 white men, and 11 slaves.
18	8 12 4 8	78 82 85 83			8	Sb & lb	✣	cl. h.	Yesterday's diarrhœa, well; 3 in the list. Gave every man who was sent ashore on duty, and in the boats, five ounces of the tincture of bark a. m. The relapsed complaint of the 16th, is a remitting fever. All the people sleep on board.
19	8 12 4 8	81 81 83 82			9	Sb & lb	✣	h. c.	One contusion added to the list; and the old contused elbow; 5 in the list. Administer'd the bark to the shorers, who are employed in wooding and watering the ship. Plenty of fish caught as usual here. Though the sun shines, it is nevertheless very hazy.
20	8 12 4 8	81 82 83 82			10	Sb & lb	✣	h. c.	The complaint of the 15th, well; and 1 contusion added to the list; 4 in it, as the contused elbow, which is become scrophulous, does the duty of a centinel. Gave the shorers the tincture of bark. Many of them got drunk last night, and 1 was left in the woods. Heavy dews, no stock to be got.

X

Year, Months, and Days.	Hours.	Thermometer	Latitude or different parts.	Longitude made.	Moon's Age	Winds.	Rain and Dew.	Appearances of the Atmosphere.	REMARKS, AND STATE OF THE SICK LIST.
1774 Feb. 21	8 12 4 8	80 82 83 80	Sierra Leon.		11	Sb & lb	❖	h. c.	No alteration in the lift. Gave the men the tincture of bark. P. m. the man came on board who was left afhore the 19th. Though he did not complain, I entered him n the fick lift.
22	8 12 8	80 82 81			12	Sb & lb	❖	h. c.	The contufion of the 19th, well; 1 feverifh complaint added to the lift, from going into the water with a profufe fweat on him; 5 in the lift. Gave the people the tincture of bark.
23	8 12 8	80 82 81			13	Sb & lb	❖	h. c.	The man who lay afhore, returned to his duty, but takes medicine, 1 feverifh complaint from the fame caufe as yefterday's added to the lift; 5 in it. The men got the tincture.
24	8 12 8	80 81 81			14	Sb & lb	❖	h. c.	The complaint of the 22d, and yefterday's well; 3 in the lift. Gave the fhorers the tincture of bark.
25	8 12 8	79 81 81			15	Sb & lb	❖	h. c.	The relapfed complaint of the 16th, well; 1 diarrhœa, 1 with feverifh fymptoms, 1 with the piles, and 1 lame complaint, added to the lift; 6 in it. The fcorbutick cafe much better from having been fent afhore every day. The men got the tincture of bark. P. m. failed.
26	8 12 4 8	80 81 82 81	08° 26″		p. a. m.	f N t NW *	❖	h. c.	Yefterday's diarrhœa has been bad this month, though he did not complain, he has a very bad fever and fevere gripes, with his purging, 1 diarrhœa from eating oyfters, added to the lift; 7 in it.
27	8 12 8	81 81 81	08° 19″	from Cape Sierra Leon 00° 32″ W	17	f WNW t NW **	❖	h.	Yefterday's diarrhœa, and the feverifh complaint of the 25th, well; 5 in the lift. A hypochondriack cafe, not in it.
28	8 12 4 8	80 81 83 f 82	08° 06″	00° 42″ W	18	f WNW t NW *	❖	h. c.	The piles of the 25th, well; 3 feverifh complaints, 1 with eruptions, and 1 cough, added to the lift; none of them were fhorers, 9 in it. 1 bad fever with a flux, 1 fcurvy, 1 lame complaint, and 1 contufion, befides them who complained this day.
Martii 1 Die Martis	8 12 8	81 83 82	07° 36″	00° 48″ W	19	V *	❖	h.	The contufion of the 20th ult. yefterday's cough, and 1 of the feverifh complaints, well; 6 in the lift befides the hypochondria who takes no medicine.
2	8 12 8	81 82 80	07° 08″	00° 02″ W	20	N Wly *	❖	h.	One feverifh complaint added to the lift; 7 in it.
3	8 12 8	80 80 81	06° 48″	00° 45″ E	21	N Wly *	❖	h.	One feverifh complaint added to the lift the 28th ult. well; they feem to proceed from a redundancy of the bile, 6 in the lift.

Year, Months, and Days.	Hours.	Thermometer.	Latitude or different parts.	Longitude made.	Moon's age.	Winds.	Rain or Dew.	Appearances of the Atmosphere.	REMARKS, AND STATE OF THE SICK LIST.
1774 Martii 4	8 12 8	81 79 80	06° 26″	01° 41″ E	22	V *	❖	cl. h.	The complaint with eruptions of the 28th, well; 5 in the lift. The fame complaint of the 25th, is an old fiftula in ano
5	8 12 8	80 78 79	06° 06″	from Cape Montferado 00° 11″ E	23	V *	❖	h.	No alteration in the lift.
6	8 12 8	79 78 80	05° 20″	01° 15″ E	24	N Wly *	❖	h.	The purging; or bad fever of the 25th ult. died—he was elderly and fubject to complaints in his bowels, and the complaint of the 2d, well; 3 in the lift.
7	8 12 8	80 80 82	04° 37″	02° 06″ E	25	Sb & lb *	❖	h.	No alteration in the lift. Off Cetera Crue, from whence very fmall canoes always come on board, the men are dextrous in fwimming and diving, and in begging I may fay.
8	8 12 4 8	81 81 82 81	04° 30″		26	Sb & lb *	❖	h.	Three in the lift. Sailing along the land.
9	8 12 8	81 83 f 81	04° 20″		27	Sb & lb *	❖	h.	No alteration in the lift. Our fails are black with mildew, from the heavy dews in the night and the fog by day, and every thing on board is quite damp and mouldy; the wood fhrinks and iron rufts amazingly. The fhip's decks are very damp too, notwithftanding the fun fhines. No perfon on board refrefhed from fleep.
10	8 12 4 8	81 81 82 81	04° 41″		28	Sb & lb *	❖	h. cl.	No alteration in the lift. Not far from the land.
11	8 12 8	81 81 80	04° 44″	from St. Andrews 00° 30″ E	29	Sb & lb *	❖	h. cl.	The other feverifh complaint of the 28th, well; in the lift. But neither the fcrophulous albe nor hypochondria are well.
12	8 12 8	79 80 80	Cape Le Hou		m. a. m.	Sb & lb *	❖	h.	One feverifh complaint added to the lift; 3 in [illegible]
13	8 12 4 8	80 81 83 81	05° 08″		2	Sb & lb *	❖	h.	Yefterday's complaint well; 2 in the lift.
14	 12 8	82 83 82	. m. Cape Appalonia 04° 50″		3	Sb & lb **	❖	cl.	No alteration in the lift. 9 A. m. anchord at Appalonia, about five miles from the fhore, and failed at 1 p. m.

Year, Months, and Days.	Hours.	Thermometer.	Latitude or different parts.	Longitude made.	Moon's age.	Winds.	Rain or Dew.	Appearances of the Atmosphere.	REMARKS, AND STATE OF THE SICK LIST.
1774 Martii 15	8 12 8	81 83 82	05° 04″ Cape Coast	02° 10″ W L. O.	4	Sb & lb	❖	c.	The same complaint of the 25th ult. does duty, though not quite well; the scorbutick case only in the list. Some slight opthalmick complaints who do duty. 1 p. m. anchored.
16	8 12 8	81 82 81			5	Sb & lb		c.	No alteration in the list. We lye about two miles from the shore.
17	8 12 8	82 82 81			6	Sb & lb		c.	One in the list only. Employed in watering the ship. The waterers get the tincture of bark in the morning. There is but little water in the pond, and that is thick. Some quick lime is therefore thrown into it; it is well strained and to be used only for boiling the provisions, and to be given to the stock. The scorbutick case sent ashore every day.
18	8 12 8	83 82 80			7	Sb & lb		cl. c.	No alteration in the list. Gave the waterers the tincture of bark. The men get a great deal of New-England new rum from the blacks, and are continually drunk.
19	8 12 4 8	80 83 84 81			8	Sb & lb		cl. c.	One in the list. Gave the waterers the tincture of bark; neither stock nor vegetables to be got worth notice.
20	8 12 8	83 83 82			9	Sb & lb		cl. c.	The list continues the same. Gave the waterers the tincture.
21	8 12 4 8	83 83 84 82			10	Sb & lb		cl. c.	No alteration in the list. Administered the tincture to the waterers. The men keep constantly drunk.
22	8 12 4 8	83 84 85 83			11	Sb & lb		cl. c.	One only in the list. Gave the waterers the tincture. The thermometer in the Castle, has not been below 82, nor higher than 86, since we arrived.
23	8 12 8	83 82 81			12	Sb & lb		cl.	The scorbutick pretty well recovered, and does some duty. 7 P. m. sailed. The people where we have touched on the coast, were all healthy generally.
24	8 12 8	81 82 82	04° 15″	from Cape Coast 00° 05″ W	13	W *		c.	The hypochondria continues bad, the scrophulous elbow rather worse, the fistulous complaint not quite well, 1 opthalmia, 1 excoriation, and 1 feverish complaint added to the list; 5 in it.
25	8 12 8	83 83 81	03° 07″	00° 26″ E	14	a. m. W p. m. SSE ⁂	. . .	cl.	No alteration in the list; only yesterday's feverish complaint has a diarrhœa.

Year, Months, and Days.	Hours.	Thermometer.	Latitude or different parts.	Longitude made.	Moon's Age	Winds.	Rain and Dew.	Appearances of the Atmosphere.	REMARKS, AND STATE OF THE SICK LIST.
1774 Martii 26	8 12 4 8	81 82 83 81	02° 10″ R.	00° 26″ E from Cape Coaſt	15	W *		cl. c.	The feveriſh complaint of the 24th, well; 4 in the liſt. Neither the ſcorbutick, who is not quite well, nor the old fiſtula in ano, are included in it.
27	8 12 8	83 82 82	01° 24″	01° 04″ E	p. p. m.	WSW SWbW *		c.	No alteration in the liſt.
28	8 12 8	81 83 82	00° 51″	01° 37″ E	17	V *	.	cl.	The liſt continues the ſame.
29	8 12 4 8	82 82 84 82	00° 37″	01° 54″ E	18	V *		cl.	Four in the liſt. Hardly an air of wind, and very ſultry.
30	8 12 8	83 83 84	00° 14″	01° 49″ E	19	EbS *	.	cl.	The opthalmia of the 24th, well; 3 in the liſt.
31	8 12 8	83 83 81	00° 18″ South	02° 37″ E	20	EbS *	p. m. . . .	cl.	No alteration in the liſt. We fell in with a New England whale fiſhing veſſel, eight months out, and only the maſter bad, of a remitting fever. I ſpared him ſome bark and other medicines which I preſcribed for him; he came on board of our ſhip. The hypochondria, the ſcrophula, and excoriation are the 3.
Aprilis 1 Die Veneris	8 12 8	81 83 82	00° 49″	02° 16″ E	21	f SbW t SbE *		cl. c.	Two fluxes, marines, added to the liſt; and 1 excoriation; 6 in it, beſides the ſcorbutick and fiſtula, who do ſome duty.
2	8 12 8	84 84 83	01° 16″	01° 33″ E	22	f SbE t SSW *	. .	cl.	Three fluxes, 2 of them marines, added to the liſt; 9 in it.
3	8 12 8	83 83 82	01° 48″	00° 16″ E	23	f SbE t SSW *	. .	cl.	No alteration in the liſt. The fluxes are very bad dyſenteries.
4	8 12 8	80 82 82	02° 16″	00° 22″ W	24	f SbE t SbW *	. .	cl.	The excoriation of the 1ſt, has got a flux. No other alteration in the liſt.
5	8 12 8	82 82 81	03° 06″	01° 44″ W	25	S SbE **		cl. c.	Yeſterday's flux well; but his excoriation not yet healed; 9 in the liſt.
6	8 12 8	82 82 82	04° 03″	03° 20″ W	26	S SbE **		c. cl.	One flux, a marine, added to the liſt; 10 in it.

Year, Months, and Days.	Hours.	Thermometer.	Latitude or different parts.	Longitude made.	Moon's age.	Winds.	Rain or Dew.	Appearances of the Atmosphere.	REMARKS, AND STATE OF THE SICK LIST.
1774 Aprilis 7	8 12 8	81 80 81	04° 37″	05°55″ W from Cape Coast	27	f SbE t SE **		c. cl.	No alteration in the list. Yesterday's flux is a dysentery. All the dysenteries are very bad.
8	8 12 8	82 80 80	04° 41″	08°09″ W	28	f SE t SbE **		c.	One old man added to the list with the scurvy, he is subject to it; 11 in it.
9	8 12 8	82 80 80	04° 48″	09°47″ W	29	f SbE t SEbS **		c.	One flux added to the list; 12 in it.
10	8 12 8	82 81 81	04° 51″	12°04″ W	m. p. m.	f SbE t SEbS **		c.	One marine a dysentery of the 1st, and the excoriation, well; 10 in the list.
11	8 12 8	81 81 81	04° 41″	14°42″ W	1	f SbE t SEbS **		cl.	One marine a dysentery, well; 9 in the list.
12	8 12 8	83 82 82	04° 34″	17°08″ W	2	SE **	.	cl.	One of the dysenteries, (a marine) added to the list the 2d, died; 8 in the list.
13	8 12 8	83 82 82	04° 25″	19°48″ W	3	f EbS t SSE **	. .	cl.	One marine took ill yesterday with the flux, but did not complain, added to the list; 9 in it.
4	8 12 8	83 83 83	04° 15″	22°42″ W	4	f EbS t SSE **		cl. c.	One dysentery added to the list; 10 in it.
15	8 12 8	83 82 82	04° 04″	25°10″ W	5	SEbE **		c. cl.	The dysentery of the 13th died, 1 old rheumatism added to the list; 10 in it.
16	8 12 8	83 82 82	03° 04″	27° 15″ W 30°00″ W L. O.	6	a. m. SEbE p. m. V *	p. m. . . .	c. cl.	Yesterday's complaint does duty; 9 in the list.
17	8 12 8	83 82 82	02° 30″ R.	28°03″ W	7	V *	. . .	cl.	One dysentery added to the list; 10 in it. Disagreeable weather.
18	8 12 8	81 81 81	02° 11″	28° 35″ W	8	f SE t NEbN **	. . . .	cl.	No alteration in the list. Very disagreeable weather.
19	8 12 8	80 79 81	01° 05″ R.	30°21″ W	9	f SE t NEbN **	. . . .	cl.	One fever, a marine, 1 dysentery, 1 griped complaint, and 1 nausea from eating shark, added to the list; 14 in it.

Year, Months, and Days.	Hours.	Thermometer.	Latitude or different parts.	Longitude made.	Moon's age.	Winds.	Rain or Dew.	Appearances of the Atmosphere.	REMARKS, AND STATE OF THE SICK LIST.
1774 Aprilis 20	8 12 8	80 80 80	00° 19″ R.	31° 32″ W	10	f SE t NEbN **	. .	cl.	Yesterday's griped complaint, and the naufea well; 12 in the lift.
21	8 12 8	81 82 82	00° 06″ North R.	32° 09″ W	11	V **	. .	cl.	One dyfentery, a marine, added to the lift; 13 in it.
22	8 12 8	82 80 81	00° 33″ R.	32° 49″ W	12	f E tNE *	. . .	cl.	One fcorbutick, who is very feverifh, added to the lift; 14 in it.
23	8 12 8	81 81 81	0° 17″	35° 10″ W	13	f E t NE *	. .	cl.	No alteration in the lift, or weather.
24	8 12 8	81 80 80	02° 23″	36° 26″ W	14	f E t NE *	. . . .	cl.	One fcurvy added to the lift; 15 in it. All the fcorbuticks are feamen.
25	8 12 8	79 79 78	03° 31″ R.	37° 34″ W	15	V ***	. . . .	cl.	One fcurvy added to the lift. P. m. the dyfentery of the 21ft, died, 15 in the lift. The dyfenteries who were recovering, grow worfe again. Very bad weather, and Squally.
26	8 12 8	79 79 80	04° 28″	38° 54″ W	p. a. m.	f NEbN t ENE **		c. cl.	One added to the lift with a naufea; 16 in it.
27	8 12 8	80 81 80	05° 57″	40° 39″ W	17	NE **	. .	cl.	The fcorbutick of the 25th does duty, though not well; 1 fever, a marine, added to the lift; 16 in it.
28	8 12 8	80 79 80	07° 20″	42° 02″ W	18	f SE t NEbN **	. .	cl.	The fever of the 19th, the complaint of the 26th and yefterday's fever, well; 1 headach added to the lift; 14 in it.
29	8 12 8	80 78 79	08° 24″ R.	43° 06″ W	19	NEbN **	. . . .	cl.	The dyfentery of the 6th, well; 1 dyfentery, and 1 griped complaint, added to the lift; 15 in it.
30	8 12 8	80 79 80	09° 27″	44° 16″ W	20	NE **		c. cl.	The dyfentery of the 17th, died, 14 in the lift.
Maii 1 Die Sabbati	8 12 8	81 81 81	10° 25″	45° 36″ W 53° 40″ W L. O.	21	NE **		c. cl.	One flux of the 2d, the flux of the 9th, the head ach of the 28th, the griped complaint of the 29th, and the excoriation of the 24th, ult. well; the old fcurvy added to the lift; 10 in it. 4 Dyfenteries, 4 fcurvies, 1 white fwelling or fcrophula, and 1 hypochondria.

Year Months and Days.	Hours.	Thermometer.	Latitude or different Parts.	Longitude made.	Moon's age.	Winds.	Rain or Dew.	Appearances of the Atmosphere.	REMARKS, AND STATE OF THE SICK LIST.
1774 Maii 2	8 12 8	81 81 81	11° 57″	47° 11″ W 54° 37″ W L O	22	NEbE **	.	c. cl.	The fcurvy who did duty the 27th, the flux of the 9th ult. who was returned well yefterday re lapfed, and 1 large fcorbutick ulcer added to the lift; 13 in it.
3	8 12 8	81 80 80	13° 55″	48°37″ W	23	ENE **		c.	Yefterday's relapfed flux, well; 1 fcurvy, and fcald, added to the lift; 14 in it.
4	8 12 8	80 80 81	15° 27″	50°06″ W	24	f SEbE t E **		c.	One fcurvy added to the lift; 15 in it. Befides fome ulcers.
5	8 12 8	80 81 81	16° 20″	51°41″ W	25	E *		c. cl.	The dyfentery of the 14th ult. well; 1 with feverifh fymptoms added to the lift; 15 in it.
6	8 12 8	80 80 81	9 a. m. Defeada 16° 39″	61°35″ W L. O.	26	E *		cl. c.	One feverifh complaint added to the lift; 16 in it. We were much out in our reckoning; (but made Defeada exactly by the lunar obfervation,) the reafon affigned for which and our having had fo rainy a paffage, is our having been carried over too far to the weftward, and thereby too near to the Spanifh main, by a current.
7	8 12 8	81 81 81	a. m. Antigua		27	Sb & lb		c. cl.	One contufion added to the lift; 17 in it. Sent the 8 fcurvies, 1 fcrophula, and 2 weak dyfenteries to the hofpital. We anchored at 8 a. m. in Freeman's bay, Englifh harbour. Not a fhip in it but our own, the admiral and fquadron being on a cruize.
8	8 12 8	82 82 81			28	Sb & lb	.	c. cl.	The complaint of the 6th, well; 5 in the lift. The men get new rum off from the fhore, and are frequently drunk.
9	8 12 8	82 82 81			29	Sb & lb	.	c. cl.	The complaint of the 5th, well; 4 in the lift. No frefh meat and few or any vegetables to be got.
10	8 12 8	82 82 81			m. p. m.	p. m. V *	.	c. cl.	Five of the fcurvies, and the fcrophula returned from the hofpital; 1 fcurvy, 1 fuppreffion of urine, and 2 fevers, one of whom was returned to duty the 8th, added to the lift; 14 in it. Sailed at m
11	8 12 8	81 81 80	a. m. St. Chriftophers		1	V **	.	c. cl.	No alteration of the lift. Anchored in old road, to water the fhip at 10 a. m. P. m. A number of the men drunk.
12	8 12 8	80 81 80			2	V **	.	c. cl.	The fuppreffion of urine of the 10th died (See the review for this month) and the contufion of the 7th, well; the headach returned well the 1ft, relapfed, and 1 fcurvy added to the lift; 14 in it.

Year, Months, and Days.	Hours.	Thermometer.	Latitude or different parts.	Longitude made.	Moon's age.	Winds.	Rain or Dew.	Appearances of the Atmosphere.	REMARKS, AND STATE OF THE SICK LIST.
1774 Maii 13	8 12 8	80 80 80			3	f NE t E **		c. cl.	The fevers of the 10th are remittents, and yesterday's headach remits. No other alteration in the lift. Sailed at 6 a. m.
14	8 12 8	80 80 80	17° 10″	from St. Chriftophers 02° 04″ W	4	f NE t E **		c. cl.	The fcald of the 4th, well; and 1 lame complaint added to the lift; 14 in it.
15	8 12 8	80 81 81	17° 08″	04° 02″ W	5	f NE t E *		c. cl.	Two fluxes, 1 was returned to duty the 5th, and 2 headachs, added to the lift; 18 in it.
16	8 12 8	81 81 81	17° 19″	06° 02″ W	6	f SEbE t ESE *		c. cl.	The dyfentery of the 29th ult. well; 17 in the lift
17	8 12 8	81 81 81	17° 23″	07° 30″ W	7	f SEbE t E *		c. cl.	The relapfed headach of the 12th, well, 1 dyfentery added to the lift; 17 in it.
18	8 12 4 8	81 81 79 81	17° 26″	from Al tavella 00° 18″ W	8	f E t SEbE	.	c. cl.	The lame complaint of the 14th, and 1 of the fluxes of the 15th well; 15 in the lift. One of the remittents of the 10th pretty well, but he has an ulcer on his leg.
19	8 12 8	78 77 79	17° 45″	01° 45″ W	9	V ***	. . . .	t. l. cl.	One feverifh complaint added to the lift; 16 in it The people being up all night from a top maft being carried away, I gave each of them a wine glafs full of tincture of bark a. m. with the Captain's approbation.
20	8 12 8	81 79 81	18° 03″	from Navaffa 00° 21″ W	10	V ***	. . .	cl.	No alteration in the lift.
21	8 12 8	81 81 82	Jamaica		11	a. m. V **		c. cl.	One of the fevers of the 10th, and the complaint of the 19th, well, 1 cough added to the lift; 15 in it. We anchored at Port Royal 5 p. m.
22	8 12 8	82 82 82			12	Sb & lb		cl.	Sent the 7 fcurvies, feamen, 2 foul ulcers, the fcrophula, and the relapfed flux of the 15th, to the hofpital; the ulcers were not in the fick lift The flux of the 17th, well; 2 dyfenteries, 1 with eruptions, and the old relapfed headach again added to the lift; 9 in it. Sir George Rodney commands here ftill. As frefh beef is allowed to the fhips only once a week, and as our men have been fo long with out any, or vegetables, and are fickly, I wrote to the Captain to apply to the admiral for frefh beef every meat day for the fhip's company, but he would only allow it us twice a week.
23	8 12 8	82 83 83			13	Sb & lb		c.	Sent a flux to the hofpital, who was not in the lift. No alteration in it.

Year, Months, and Days.	Hours.	Thermometer	Latitude or different parts.	Longitude made.	Moon's Age	Winds.	Rain and Dew.	Appearances of the Atmosphere.	REMARKS, AND STATE OF THE SICK LIST.
1774 Maii 24	8 12 8	82 82 83	Jamaica		14	Sb & lb		c. cl.	Nine in the lift. The men get very drunk with new rum.
25	8 12 8	82 83 83			p. p. m.	Sb & lb ***		c. cl.	One of the dyfenteries of the 22d, fent to the hofpital, a marine, and the relapfed headach well; 7 in the lift.
26	8 12 4 8	82 85 86 85			16	Sb ***		c. cl.	Sent the other dyfentery of the 22d, and the cough of the 21ft to the hofpital, and the complaint with eruptions of the 22d well, 1 flux, and 1 with a pain in his ftomach added to the lift; 6 in it. Very hot.
27	8 12 8	83 84 84			17	Sb & lb		c.	No alteration in the lift.
28	8 12 8	82 85 84			18	Sb & lb		c.	One added to the lift, with feverifh fymptoms; 7 in it.
29	8 12 8	81 85 84			19	Sb & lb		c. cl.	One of the headachs of the 15th, and the pain of the ftomach of the 26th, well; 1 dyfentery, and 1 fever, marines, added to the lift; 7 in it.
30	8 12 8	82 84 84			20	Sb & lb		c. cl.	Sent the fever of the 28th, and both yefterday's complaints to the hofpital; 4 in the lift.
31	8 12 8	82 85 84			21	Sb & lb	.	c. cl.	The other headach of the 15th, and the dyfentery of the 26th, well; 2 added to the lift with feverifh fymptoms. The hypochondria, the remittent of the 10th. now an ulcer, and this day's complaints, are the 4 in the lift.
Junii 1 Die Mercurii	8 12 8	82 84 83			22	Sb **	.	c. cl.	Two with feverifh fymptoms, 1 dyfentery, and the old relapfing remitting headach, now become hectick, added to the lift; 8 in it. Some of the fcorbuticks in the hofpital are feized with the dyfentery from being in the fame ward with the dyfenteries
2	8 12 8	83 83 83			23	Sb **	.	c. cl.	The hectick complaint, and yefterday's dyfentery fent to the hofpital; 6 in the lift.
3	8 12 8	83 83 83			24	Sb **		c. cl.	One foul ulcer, now entered from a Guinea fhip, added to the lift; 7 in it. One of the feverifh complaints of the 31ft ult. is a dyfentery.
4	8 12 8	81 85 84			25	Sb & lb		c. cl.	Sent the dyfentery mentioned yefterday to the hofpital. The marine, a dyfentery fent there the 30th ult. died.

Year, Months, and Days.	Hours.	Thermometer.	Latitude or different Parts.	Longitude made.	Moon's age.	Winds.	Rain or Dew.	Appearances of the Atmosphere.	REMARKS, AND STATE OF THE SICK LIST.
1774 Junii 5	8 12 4 8	83 84 85 84	Jamaica		26	Sb **		c. cl	The other fever of the 1ſt, well; 5 in the liſt. The people continue to get drunk.
6	8 12 8	82 85 83			27	Sb **		c. cl.	The other feveriſh complaint of the 31ſt, well; 4 in it.
7	8 12 4 8	83 84 85 84			28	Sb **		c. cl.	No alteration in the liſt.
8	8 12 4 8	83 85 86 84			29	Sb & lb		c. cl.	One diarrhœa from drunkenneſs added to the liſt 5 in it.
9	8 12 8	83 85 84			m. a. m.	Sb **		c. cl.	Yeſterday's complaint well; 4 in the liſt.
10	8 12 4 8	83 85 86 84			2	Sb **		c. cl.	No alteration in the liſt. Some ſlight drunken complaints, but not in the liſt.
11	8 12 8	83 85 84			3	Sb **		c.	One feveriſh complaint well; 3 in liſt.
12	8 12 8	83 85 84			4	Sb **		c.	Three in the liſt.
3	8 12 8	83 85 84			5	Sb **		c. cl.	The ulcer of the 3d, ſent to the hoſpital; 2 in the liſt.
14	8 12 8	84 85 84			6	Sb & lb		c.	No alteration in the liſt.
15	8 12 8	81 84 82			7	Sb & lb		c.	Two in the liſt.
16	8 12 8	82 85 83			8	Sb & lb		c.	No alteration in the liſt.

Year, Months, and Days.	Hours.	Thermometer.	Latitude or different parts.	Longitude made.	Moon's age.	Winds.	Rain or Dew.	Appearances of the Atmofphere.	REMARKS, AND STATE OF THE SICK LIST.
1774 Junii 17	8 12 8	81 83 83	Jamaica		9	Sb & lb		c.	The marine catarrhous cough of the 28th of December is become fcorbutick, and fent to the hofpital; he had a very bad fever and continued long weak after it; 2 in the lift.
18	8 12 8	80 84 83			10	Sb & lb		c.	One remitting fever fent to fick quarters, he was took ill the 16th, though he did not complain; 2 in the lift.
19	8 12 8	81 84 83			11	Sb & lb		c.	No alteration in the lift.
20	8 12 8	80 85 83			12	Sb & lb		c.	No alteration in the lift. It is a little cloudy fometimes.
21	8 12 8	81 84 82			13	Sb & lb		c.	One dyfentery complained and was fent to the hofpital. The lift continues the fame.
22	8 12 8	81 84 83			14	Sb & lb		c.	One lame complaint, and 1 with feverifh fymptoms, added to the lift; 4 in it.
23	8 12 8	82 84 83			p. p. m.	Sb & lb		c.	One headach added to the lift; 5 in it.
24	8 12 8	81 84 82			16	Sb & lb		c.	The complaints of the 22d, well; 3 in the lift.
25	8 12 8	81 83 81			17	Sb & lb		c.	The headach of the 23d, well; and 1 contufion added to the lift; 3 in it.
26	8 12 8	81 84 82			18	Sb & lb		c.	Yefterday's contufion fent to the hofpital, and 1 wound added to the lift; 3 in it.
27	8 12 8	82 84 83			19	Sb & lb		c.	No alteration in the lift. Admiral Gayton arrived in His Majefty's Ship Antelope.
28	8 12 8	81 84 82			20	Sb & lb		c.	Three in the lift. The remittent fent the 18th, returned well from fick quarters.
29	8 12 8	81 83 83			21	Sb & lb		c.	No alteration in the lift. One marine, a flux, died at the hofpital.

Year, Months, and Day.	Hours.	Thermometer	Latitude or different parts.	Longitude made.	Moon's Age	Winds.	Rain and Dew.	Appearances of the Atmosphere.	REMARKS, AND STATE OF THE SICK LIST.
1774 Junii 30	8 12 8	80 84 83	Jamaica		22	Sb & lb		c.	Three in the lift. The hypochondria, the ulcer, and the wound of the 26th.
Julii 1 Die Veneris	8 12 8	81 84 83			23	Sb & lb		c.	No alteration in the lift.
2	8 12 8	80 84 83			24	Sb & lb	.	c. cl.	One with feverifh fymptoms added to the lift; in it.
3	8 12 8	80 83 83			25	Sb & lb		c.	One feverifh complaint from drunkennefs, added to the lift; 5 in it.
4	8 12 4 8	80 83 84 83			26	Sb & lb	.	c. cl.	The complaint of the 2d, well; and 1 drunker feverifh complaint added to the lift.
5	8 12 8	80 83 83			27	Sb & lb		c.	The complaint of the 3d, well; 4 in the lift.
6	8 12 8	81 85 84			28	Sb & lb		c.	No alteration in the lift. A little cloudy at times
7	8 12 8	81 82 80			29	Sb & lb	. .	c. cl.	The complaint of the 4th, well; 3 in the lift
8	8 12 8	81 86 84			m. p. m.	Sb & lb	.	cl.	No alteration in the lift.
9	8 12 8	81 85 84			1	Sb & lb		c.	One feverifh complaint added to the lift; 4 in it. P. m. the fick people were brought off from the hofpital; but the hectick cafe was fo weak, from a dyfentery, that he was left there; 7 invalids fent from thence on board of us.
10	8 12 8	81 85 83			2	Sb & lb		c.	The ulcer well. Some of the men who came laft night from the hofpital are worfe than when they were fent to it; 9 of them are added to the lift; 12 in it; 1 hypochondria, 1 dyfentery, 1 epilepfy, he was fent a dyfentery the 22d May, 1 valetudinarian flux, 4 fcorbutick fluxes, 1 fcrophula, 1 contufion, 1 wound, and 1 feverifh complaint. The invalids are 1 blind of an eye, 1 gout, 1 with obftructions in the abdomen, from a remitting fever, 1 headach from an old fracture of the cranium, 1 very large foul ulcer, and 2 valetudinarians, fluxes.

Year, Months, and Days.	Hours.	Thermometer.	Latitude or different Parts.	Longitude made.	Moon's age.	Winds.	Rain or Dew.	Appearances of the Atmosphere.	REMARKS, AND STATE OF THE SICK LIST.
1774 Julii 11	8 12 8	81 85 84	Jamaica		3	Sb & lb		cl.	One with a naufea added to the lift; 13 in it.
12	8 12 8	81 84 82	Sailed a. m.		4	Sb **	. .	cl.	Yefterday's complaint well ; 12 in the lift. Six a. m. failed with Sir Geo. Rodney on board of the Portland.
13	8 12 8	80 83 83	Off Jamaica		5	f ESE t ENE **	. .	cl. c.	One lame complaint added to the lift; 13 in it.
14	8 12 8	83 83 83	18° 31″	from Port Royal 00° 45″ W	6	f ESE t ENE **	.	cl. c.	One of the fcorbutick fluxes, took ill the 21ft ult. well; 12 in the lift.
15	8 12 8	84 84 83	18° 48″		7	f ESE t ENE **	. .	cl. c.	One griped complaint added to the lift; 13 in it.
16	8 12 8	83 84 83	18° 18″	from Point Morant 00° 37″ W	8	f ESE t ENE *		c. cl.	The feverifh complaint of the 9th, well; and contufion added to the lift; 13 in it.
17	8 12 8	83 83 83	18° 23″ Navaffa		9	f ESE tENE*** p. m.		c. cl.	One of the fcorbutick fluxes, took ill the 12th of May with the fcurvy, and the complaint of the 15th, well; 11 in the lift.
18	8 12 4 8	83 83 85 83	18° 44″ Cape Dona Maria		10	f ESE t ENE **	. .	cl. c.	The lame complaint of the 13th, and the contufion of the 16th; well; 9 in the lift.
19	8 12 8	83 84 83	18° 44″		11	f ESE t ENE **		cl. c.	One of the fcorbutick fluxes, took ill the 3d of May with the fcurvy, and the wound of the 25th ult. well; 1 lame complaint added to the lift; 8 in it.
20	8 12 4 8	84 84 85 84	18° 58″		12	f ESE t ENE **		c. cl.	One of the hofpital fcorbuticks feized with a nervous fever. No other alteration in the lift.
21	8 12 4 8	84 85 87 85	19° 31″ Off Cape Nicholas		13	SSE **		c. cl.	The marine a fcorbutick flux, and the lame complaint of the 19th, well; 6 in the lift. Four of the invalids do fome duty. An exceeding hot day.
22	8 12 8	85 85 84	19° 55″ Cape Nicholas Mole		14	ENE *		c.	No alteration in the lift. Anchored with the Portland in the mole. There is a large town built here, fince the late war, with which the Americans carry on a great trade.

Year, Months, and Days.	Hours.	Thermometer.	Latitude or different parts.	Longitude made.	Moon's age.	Winds.	Rain or Dew.	Appearances of the Atmosphere.	REMARKS, AND STATE OF THE SICK LIST.
1774 Julii 23	8 12 8	83 85 83			15	Sb & lb		c.	The hospital dysentery, well; 5 in the list. Pretty good water here. Getting some on board.
24	8 12 4 8	82 84 85 83			p. a. m.	Sb & lb		c.	One belly-ach added to the list; 6 in it.
25	8 12 8	82 84 85	19° 56″		17	f NNE t E *		c.	Yesterday's complaint well; 5 in it. Sailed with the Portland a. m.
26	8 12 8	82 83 83	20° 48″ Hispaniola		18	E **		c. cl.	No alteration in the list.
27	8 12 8	83 82 82	20° 42″ Heniago		19	f E t NE **		cl.	Five in the list.
28	8 12 4 8	83 83 84 83	21° 16″ Heniago		20	f EbS t NE *** a. m.		c. cl.	No alteration in the list. I discovered the contusion of the 25th ult. to be a fracture of the head of the *os femoris*. I was not on board when it happened, and it was never suspected at the hospital.
29	8 12 8	83 83 82	22° 29″	from Mayguana 00° 11″ E	21	EbN *		c.	One headach added to the list; 6 in it.
30	8 12 8	84 84 83	23° 26″	00° 11″ E	22	EbN *		c.	Yesterday's headach well; 5 in the list.
31	8 12 8	83 83 82	24° 09″	00° 11″ E	23	f EbN t SE *		c.	No alteration in the list. The hypochondria, the Epilepsy, the nervous fever, the scrophula, and 1 contusion, are the 5 in it. Four of the invalids do some duty.
Aug. 1 Die Lunæ	8 12 8	83 83 83	25° 31″	00° 41″ E	24	f SE t SSE **		c. cl.	No alteration in the list.
2	8 12 8	83 83 83	26° 51″	02° 25″ E	25	f SE t SSE **		c. cl.	Five in the list. A little cloudy at times, and very warm.
3	8 12 8	83 83 82	27° 51″	03° 45″ E	26	f SEbE t SbE **	.	c. cl.	Five in the list.
4	8 12 8	83 83 82	28° 43″	05° 10″ E	27	f SEbE t SbE **		c. cl.	The list continues the same.

Year, Months, and Days.	Hours.	Thermometer.	Latitude or different parts.	Longitude made.	Moon's age.	Winds.	Rain or Dew.	Appearances of the Atmosphere.	REMARKS, AND STATE OF THE SICK LIST.
1774 Aug. 5	8 12 8	82 82 79	29° 42″	06° 51″ E	28	f WNW t SbW **	. .	cl.	No alteration in the list.
6	8 12 8	81 80 79	30° 33″	08° 12″ E	29	f SSE t WSW **	. .	cl. c.	One contusion added to the list; 6 in it.
7	8 12 8	80 81 80	31° 39″	from Mayguana 10° 16″ E	m. m.	f SbE t WSW **		c. cl.	One remitting fever, an old complaint, and 1 rheumatism, added to the list; 8 in it.
8	8 12 8	81 81 81	32° 09″	12° 04″ E	2	f SSW t SbE *		c.	No alteration in the list.
9	8 12 8	81 81 80	33° 13″	12° 34″ E	3	f EbS t SEbE *		c.	The contusion of the 6th, well; 7 in the list
10	8 12 8	81 80 81	34° 25″	13° 19″ E	4	f ESE t S *		c.	No alteration in the list.
11	8 12 4 8	81 81 82 81	35° 19″	14° 43″ E	5	fS t SW **		c.	One old cough, added to the list with feverish symptoms; 8 in it.
12	8 12 8	80 80 81	36° 09″	16° 54″ E	6	SW **	.	c. cl.	No alteration in the list.
13	8 12 8	80 80 80	37° 15″	18° 58″ E	7	fSW t WSW **		c.	Eight in the list.
14	8 12 8	80 80 79	38° 16″	22° 02″ E	8	f WSW t NW **		c.	The nervous fever, well, and 1 with gripes added to the list; 8 in it. Only 3 of the invalids do duty.
15	8 12 8	79 79 80	38° 38″	24° 03″ E	9	f WSW t NW **	.	c. cl.	No alteration in the list.
16	8 12 8	76 74 75	39° 22″	27° 32″ E	10	f NW t NNW **	.	c. cl.	The remittent of the 7th, and the griped complaint of the 14th, well; 2 contusions added to the list; 8 in it.
17	8 12 8	73 70 73	39° 46″	31° 13″ E	11	f N t NNW **	.	c. cl.	The complaint of the 11th, well; and 1 headach added to the list; 8 in it. Cold weather.

Year, Months, and Days.	Hours.	Thermometer.	Latitude or different parts.	Longitude made.	Moon's age.	Winds.	Rain or Dew.	Appearances of the Atmosphere.	REMARKS, AND STATE OF THE SICK LIST.
1774 Aug. 18	8 12 8	73 73 75	40° 36″	from Mayguana 34° 36″ E	12	f N t NWbN **		c. cl.	One wound added to the list; 9 in it.
19	8 12 8	74 72 74	41° 25″	37° 20″ E	13	f N t NWbN **		c. cl.	One of the contusions of the 16th, and the head-ach of the 17th, well; 1 rheumatism added to the list; 8 in it.
20	8 12 8	74 74 73	43° 13″	40° 27″ E	14	f WSW t WNW **	.	cl.	No alteration in the list.
21	8 12 8	72 72 72	44° 19″ R.	42° 20″ E	p. p. m.	f SSE t EbS *	. .	cl. h.	Eight in the list. Disagreeable weather.
22	8 12 8	71 71 71	45° 33″ R.	43° 23″ E	16	SEbS **	.	cl. h.	No alteration in the list.
23	8 12 8	71 69 70	46° 38″	45° 42″ E	17	V *	. .	c. h.	Eight in the list.
24	8 12 8	67 66 66	47° 20″ R.	48° 13″ E	18	f WbS t NbW **	.	cl. h.	The other contusion of the 16th, well; and 2 added to the list with the rheumatism; 9 in it.
25	8 12 8	65 65 64	48° 50″	52° 16″ E	19	f NW t WNW **	.	cl.	One intermittent added to the list, he formerly had a remittent fever; 10 in the list.
26	8 12 4 8	62 62 65 63	49° 18″	56° 47″ E	20	f NW t WNW ***	.	cl. c.	No alteration in the list.
27	8 12 4 8	61 63 66 64	49° 22″	61° 10″ E	21	f NWbW t WSW ***	.	cl.	The 2 rheumatisms of the 24th, well; 8 in the list.
28	8 12 4 8	61 62 65 63	49° 28″	65° 28″ E	22	WNW ***	.	cl.	The rheumatism of the 6th, well; 7 in the list. Very cold.
29	8 12 8	61 62 63	a. m. Lands end		23	f NNW t SW **	.	cl.	The intermittent of the 25th, well; 6 in the list.

Bb

Year, Months, and Days.	Hours.	Thermometer	Latitude or different parts.	Longitude made.	Moon's Age	Winds.	Rain and Dew.	Appearances of the Atmosphere.	REMARKS, AND STATE OF THE SICK LIST.
1774 Aug. 30	8 12 8	64 6 65	49° 07″		24	W ****	.	cl. h.	One ſcald, 1 rheumatiſm, and 1 contuſion added to the liſt; 9 in it.
31	8 12 8	63 66 65	10 a. m Spithead		25	W ***	.	cl. h.	One cold added to the liſt; 10 in it.
Sept. 1 Die Veneris	8 12 8	64 67 66			26	W	.	cl. h.	Sent the epilepſy, the ſcrophulous arm, the fractured *os femoris*, and the 7 invalids, to the hoſpital. The hypochondria to go to ſick quarters. Remain in the ſick liſt, the wound of the 18th, the rheumatiſm of the 19th, the complaints of the 30th, and 31ſt ult. THE END OF THE METEOROLOGICAL JOURNAL.

PART III.

The Monthly Review of the Sick Liſt.

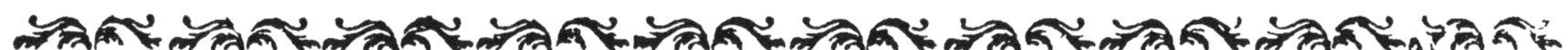

CHAPTER I.

REVIEW OF THE SICK LIST, WITH PRACTICAL OBSERVATIONS FROM THE 30th OF DECEMBER 1771, TO THE 26th OF AUGUST 1772.

IN the following review of the ſick liſt it is to be obſerved, 1ſt, That an account of the ſtate of the weather is purpoſely omitted to avoid repetitions, as that is already ſet forth at length in the meteorological journal; whereto every perſon will naturally I ſuppoſe have recourſe. 2dly, That when any diſeaſe changed to another, the patient is re-entered upon the ſick liſt under the laſt, as if he had been a freſh patient: which is to be remembered likewiſe in reading the remarks on the ſtate of the ſick liſt in the journal; and at the ſame time the two following obſervations muſt then be remembered. 3dly, That all ſlight fevers, coughs or indiſpoſitions which occured in a cold climate, are generally termed colds. 4thly, That all ſlight fevers, headachs, nauſeæ, and diarrhœæ which occurred in a hot climate, are frequently called bilious complaints, or indiſpoſitions.

DECEMBER and JANUARY, 1771-2.

The complaints that were in the ſick liſt when we ſailed, proceeded chiefly from drunkenneſs; their lying about the decks afterwards and ſleeping in their clothes: conſequently were attended with quick and full pulſes, headachs and thirſt; which were carried off by moderate bleeding, vomits, purges, the ſaline mixture, ſee p. 17. or from five and twenty to forty drops of Huxham's eſſence of antimony, given evening and morning with ſage tea or barley water for drink,

 and

and abſtinence from ſalt meat. When a cough attended the fever, a ſpermaceti or oily mixture was preſcribed, after evacuations had been made.

The contuſions, unleſs they were violent—when it became neceſſary to uſe evacuations at firſt—were cured by epithems, ſuch as oxycrate, ol. terebinth, linim. ſapon. ſp. vin. rect. camph. and compreſſes and bandages.

With reſpect to the obſervations on the method in which I preſcribed for the rheumatiſm, they are ſubjoined to the monthly review.

We had no ſooner got into a hot climate than bilious complaints made their appearance, which ſhall be taken notice of next month.

The number on the ſick liſt varied frequently, but decreaſed towards the end of the month. The diſeaſes were eleven colds with ſlight fevers, pains and coughs, five bilious indiſpoſitions, two rheumatiſms, three contuſions, and one ulcer.

February 1772.

It is worthy of obſervation, that when we anchored on the 2d of the month in Praya Bay, in the Iſland of St. Jago, there was only one patient with an ulcer in the ſick liſt; that a remitting fever made its appearance that very night—the ſentinel poſted over the water upon the booms having been taken ill of a bad fever then, and that two more were taken ill the day following with the ſame fever; after which the ſick liſt increaſed daily with bilious and remitting complaints. Whether thoſe men were actually infected from our being ſo near to the ſickly Dutch Eaſt India ſhip or not, I cannot poſitively ſay, although I am inclined to think that they were, for two reaſons, Firſt, becauſe the miaſma of infectious diſeaſes are wafted by winds to a much greater diſtance from diſeaſed bodies, than there was between the ſickly Dutch ſhip, and ours. Second, becauſe a number of the officers and ſeamen of the Rainbow, perceived at particular times, when they were looking towards the Dutch ſhip, a very diſagreeable ſmell. It was farther obſerved, that that circumſtance occurred when either our own, or the Dutch Ship veered with the wind, in ſuch a manner, as that our ſhip was to the leeward of her.

Our men had no communication with them, that having been carefully prevented by Captain Collingwood's particular directions. Whether it be doubtful or not, that the men were infected from our lying ſo cloſe to that ſickly ſhip, the caution of changing a healthy ſhip's birth, when they find themſelves near to ſo dangerous a neighbour, will moſt probably compenſate for the trouble of getting the anchor up again, and moving to a greater diſtance from her.

The lancet was cautiouſly uſed in curing the fever. Gentle emetics, and cathartics, the ſaline mixture and antimonials, cooling and ſubacid drink bee

page

page 17 and 18—and the bark with very light diet, reſtored them to health.* Some of the ſlighteſt caſes were cured as the bilious complaints, with an emetic of the tart. emetic. a doſe of ſalts the day after; Huxham's eſſence of antimony given twice a day; drink acidulated moſt commonly with lime juice or tamarinds; an abſtemious diet—ſee part IV. chap. 1. end of § 5. the elixir vitr. afterwards, forenoon and afternoon, to brace up their relaxed ſtomachs. The patients with the diarrhœæ, took 15 grains of ipecacoan. to vomit them. The other complaints were very eaſily carried off.

We had hardly got over this fever, bef re another commenced amongſt the men, who were the watering party at Sierra Leon. The ſituation they lay in aſhore, I have already deſcribed. It likewiſe appears from the journal—begun at February 27th, 1772—that none of the ſhip's company, beſides thoſe men and a man that came from a merchant ſhip, were ſeized with that fever. I therefore think it cannot admit of a doubt, that their lying aſhore was the ſole cauſe of their ſickneſs, which ſhall be ſpoken more of at large in next month's review.

The ſick liſt increaſed until the 15th day of the month, decreaſed until the 19th, and afterwards increaſed. The patients were 6 remitting fevers, 12 ſlight fevers, 2 diarrhœæ, 1 nauſea, 1 belly-ach, 2 with eruptions, 1 cough, 1 with a deafneſs, 1 contuſion, and 1 lame.

MARCH 1772.

The ſick liſt varied frequently, but rather increaſed to the 25th of the month, and then decreaſed. The diſeaſes were 6 remitting fevers, 7 ſlight fevers, 4 headachs, 4 belly-achs, 3 diarrhœæ, 1 nauſea, 1 eryſipelas 1 piles, 2 abſceſſes, 1 guinea worm, and 1 lame patient.

The remitting fever of this month was of a much more malignant nature than that at St. Jago. The paroxyſms were longer, the ſymptoms more violent, and the remiſſions leſs diſtinct. I was obliged to give either wine, tinct. cort. peruv. or tinct. theb. along with the bark, to enable the ſtomach to retain it; and to apply bliſters. Two patients only were bled; the man who came from the merchant ſhip, and a marine, who I learned was ſubject to maniacal complaints. Excepting this man, no perſon who had the remitting fever, hitherto bore that operation well, or ſeemed to receive any benefit from it; though all of them but one marine recovered within the month. See part IV. chap. 1. § 6.

The belly-achs were cured by repeated purges of the common purging ſalts, demulcent drink, thin rice or water gruel, and barley water, and ſmall doſes of opium.

The

* See the two firſt caſes of the remitting fever, Part IV. chap. 1. § 6.

The eryſipelas (the patient who came from a merchant ſhip) was cured by fomentations, cataplaſms, and ſuch medicines as relieved the bilious complaints. Thoſe ſeemed to proceed from the heat of the climate, their eating plenty of freſh fiſh, green plantains and bananas, and new fiery ſpirits which the blacks ſold them. They were cured as thoſe of laſt month.

April, 1772.

This month was yet more remarkable than any of the former, for remitting fevers; and what deſerves particular attention concerning them, is, that except one patient, they attacked thoſe men only, who ſlept aſhore at St. Thomas' iſland, the night of the great Tornado.——See the journal, page 33.—In ſeveral patients, the fever was far more malignant than it was in any of the preceding months. The paroxyſms being extremely violent; and the remiſſions very imperfect, and of ſhort duration. The fever aſſumed different types in every period. The fear of their dying, and their deſpondency were particularly diſtreſſing.

In curing it, not a man was let blood of—See part IV. chap. 1. § 6. caſe 7.

Bilious indiſpoſitions were numerous, and commenced with great violence in ſeveral patients. However, they all terminated favourably in a few days, by the ſimple method already mentioned, page 96 and 97.

The aſthmatic patient had been long ill, and came on board from the Weaſel, purpoſely to be longer in a warm climate. He had an habitual ague too, which the bark always carried off, after a vomit and purge were adminiſtered. None of the other complaints were difficult to remove.

The ſick liſt varied frequently in number. At the end of the month it was much increaſed. The patients were 10 remitting fevers, 4 ſlight fevers, 9 headachs, 2 nauſeæ, 5 diarrhœæ, 1 belly-ach, 2 from a ſuppreſſed perſpiration, 1 aſthma, 1 cough, 3 contuſions, 1 guinea worm, and 1 lame.

May, 1772.

In the beginning of the month we continued to feel the unhappy effects of the people's having ſlep aſhore at the iſland of St. Thomas, a number of them being ſeized with the fever. It is ſomewhat remarkable that none of the officers who lay aſhore that night had fevers, notwithſtanding there was no apparent material difference in their ſituations. For though they were in different parts of the houſe, they all had large wood fires. Some of them indeed had bilious complaints, and were much afraid of being taken with the fever.

I perſiſted in the ſame method of curing the fever which I had followed hitherto, and fortunately all the patients recovered but one, who died the 5th of the month, on the 7th day of his illneſs. He did not ſleep aſhore, but was much expoſed to the ſun in a boat for ſome days at that iſland. His fever never remitted,

remitted, and he was remarkably oppreſſed with fear from the moment he was ſeized. See the firſt anomalous caſe, part IV. ch. 1. § 3. I tried moderate evacuations repeatedly; the ſaline mixture with antimonials, the pediluvium, camphor, contrayerva, and bliſters. I did not adminiſter the bark, although I wiſh that I had done it, notwithſtanding the fever did not remit; and though there never appeared any indication of ſuch imminent danger, far leſs of ſuch a ſpeedy and fatal termination of it.

About the letter end of the month, ſeveral men who had been very ill of the fever, relapſed after we got into the NE trade. See the journal, page 36 and 37, where I have ſtiled thoſe relapſes, intermittents, becauſe there were real intermiſſions between the paroxyſms. The fever was in fact the ſame as that which they had had before, with the difference, that it only appeared now in a milder form. After adminiſtering an emetic and a purge, it was ſoon carried off by the bark.

The number on the ſick liſt varied ſeveral times, but decreaſed greatly towards the end of the month. The diſeaſes in all were 4 remitting fevers, 4 relapſed fevers, 5 ſlight fevers, 1 head-ach, 1 nauſea, 2 coughs, 1 aſthma, and 1 hæmorrhoids.

June, 1772.

The direful conſequence of that abominable practice, which ſeamen always have of injuring their conſtitutions, by getting drunk as often as they are able to get any thing that will make them ſo; and their particular fondneſs of new ſpirits, we here experienced. See the journal. Thus fatally bent they are upon their own deſtruction, notwithſtanding the pain alſo of the puniſhment which they are ſure to ſuffer for their drunken riots. Some of the weakeſt of the convaleſcents from the fever likewiſe coutinued to relapſe, a few of whom were ſent to the hoſpital for the benefit of freſh diet, as the ſhip's company were allowed freſh beef only once a week. One man was killed by a fall from the main top maſt head, upon the quarter deck. No wound appeared about him, but in one of his legs, which was broke in two places. He breathed only a few minutes, though a vein was opened in each arm, and every method taken to reſtore his ſenſes. None of the other accidents were dangerous. They were cured after the ſame manner as the contuſions, page 96. Common dreſſings were applied to the wound. I preſcribed for the bilious patients, as in the month of February, page 97. The obſervations on ulcers in general are ſubjoined to the monthly review.

The ſick liſt rather increaſed all the month; the complaints of which were 1 remitting fever, 1 relapſed fever, 10 ſlight fevers; 3 headachs, 4 diarrhœæ, 1 belly-ach, 1 ſuppreſſed perſpiration, 1 eryſipelas, 1 old aſthma, 1 rheumatiſm.

 1 lumbago

1 lumbago, 7 contusions, 1 wound, 1 fracture, 1 inflammation, 1 ulcer, and 2 lame. The fracture was the man who was killed by the fall.

July, 1772.

The pernicious effects of the new rum were still manifest amongst the people: happily for them we sailed early in the month from Jamaica, and of all the bilious complaints one only, who was a hard drinker, became a remitting fever. I prescribed for them as for similar cases in the preceding months. The Guinea worm which broke, formed a large abscess, and became very troublesome, though great care was taken of it. A garlick poultice is esteemed the best application, on the coast of Africa, for extracting the worm, both before and after it is broke. Before that accident happens, the poultice certainly facilitates a more speedy extraction of the worm; but afterwards, it seems to possess no specific property in curing it. The acute pain which follows the breaking of the worm, from the inflammation, besides the trouble of dressing the parts afterwards, ought to inculcate great care to guard against pulling it out rashly; for the part is very easily healed up, if the worm be got out entire. Of the Hæmoptosis, particular notice shall be taken next month.

The sick list varied frequently in number. At the end of the month it was much decreased. All the diseases were 1 remitting fever, 5 slight fevers, 2 nauseæ, 1 diarrhœa, 1 hæmoptosis, 1 cough, 1 rheumatism, 1 contusion, 2 inflammations, and 1 Guinea worm.

August, 1772.

Fewer men complained this, than in any month of the voyage. Three only were added to the sick list before the 10th, viz. a fever, a cough, and a furuncle. The weather beginning then to be very cold, especially to them who were ill provided for it, from having sold their clothes in the West Indies for rum; most of such men were consequently seised with feverish symptoms, from the perspiration being suppressed. These complaints were soon carried off by moderate evacuations, and supplying them with clothes. The other patients were mostly soon recovered by the methods before mentioned.

The fever which was added to the sick list, the first day of the month, was anomalous, and died the 13th. He had been long drooping, and had not eat his victuals regularly. For a particular account of the case, see part IV. ch. 1. § 3. Repeated evacuations, antimonials, doctor James's fever powder, camphor, tinct. serp. virg. pulv. contrayerv. co. confect. cordiac. wine and blisters, were tried with drink.

The hæmoptosis died the 2d of the month, of the ninth severe paroxysm of his illness. He was about fourteen years of age, very weakly, and was subject to a cough, with complaints in his breast from an old hurt. The hæmoptosis began

began with a fit of coughing. In the firſt paroxyſms large quantities of black and grumous blood was thrown up; but it became gradually thinner, florid, and ſpumous. The ſtool which he had after the firſt paroxyſm, was ſomewhat bloody. His ſtools and urine contained very little or no blood ever after; and in the intermiſſions he ſpit up very little with his cough. From his being at firſt ſeized he became much dejected, and had always a degree of fever upon him. During the time of his vomiting he found great pain in his breaſt, and never complained of any pain in it at any other time; nor could he ever tell before hand that a fit was coming on. The night before he died, he was ſeized with an acute pain over one of his eyes, of which he was blind, but did not continue long. His appetite never failed him, and he ſlept very well all the time he was bad, unleſs a paroxyſm happened in the night.

By veneſection repeated in ſmall quantities, gentle purges, refrigerating and aſtringent medicines, and an abſtemious diet, there was at one time a deceitful appearance of his getting better.

When the ſhip arrived at Spithead the 26th of the month, there was only one patient, a rheumatiſm, in the ſick liſt; ſo that it rather decreaſed all the month. In all there were added to the ſick liſt, 1 remitting fever, 10 ſlight fevers, 2 headachs, 2 coughs, 1 rheumatiſm, 2 contuſions, 1 inflammation, and 1 abſceſs.

During the voyage, two patients with anomalous fevers, one with an hæmoptoſis, and one by an accident, died.

I think it well worthy of obſervation, that of all the remitting fevers that happened in the voyage, not one hepatick complaint enſued; which is a ſufficient encomium on the bark, as a cure for thoſe fevers.

CHAPTER II.

Review of the Sick List, with Practcal Observations from the 30th of November 1772, to the 24th of August, 1773.

December, 1772.

WHEN we left England, there was a number of complaints in the ſick liſt, which chiefly proceeded from intemperance before we ſailed; nor did the effects thereof ceaſe before the end of the month.

I ought

I ought to have first obferved, that while the fhip continued in England, the fhip's company was generally healthy, notwithftanding all their irregularities. In the latter end of October, three men were fent to the hofpital with very bad fevers. The headach attending them was violent, and a delirium came on very early, with a languid pulfe. 5 fevers, 2 fcurvies, 1 headach, 1 cough, 1 weak, 1 rheumatifm, 1 fuffufion, 11 Ulcers, 1 wound, and 1 lame, were fent to the hofpital in that time.

The change of climate made very little alteration on the people's health all the month, as appears in the journal: Therefore as the colds proceeded from drunkennefs, and occurred early in the month, they bore the letting blood to advantage; which together with emetics, cathartics, gentle diaphoretics, abftinence from falt provifions, and diluting drinks, foon removed them. See page 95.

The remitting fever was accompanied with a very bad cough; and as the fymptoms indicated a neceffity for it, I took away fome blood twice, and then followed the method of cure as mentioned in page 97. He recovered in fixteen days.

The intermittent was eafily cured by a vomit, a purge, and the bark, though he had often relapfed with eafterly winds. He was a brown Creole, and had a very bad remitting fever the preceding voyage, from lying afhore at the ifland of St. Thomas, fee part IV. ch. 1. § 6.

The quinfey and parotis were carried off by the fame means as the colds. The fore throat proceeded from a venereal caufe. After proper applications were made to the fractured clavicle, the patient was treated as one of the colds. Purges and an abftemious diet cured the eruptions.

The chirurgical patients were managed as fimilar cafes on the preceding voyage. The fick lift varied frequently in number. At the end of the month it contained only two patients; they were in all, 1 remitting fever, 1 intermitting fever, 1 flight fever, 7 colds with feverifh fymptoms, 2 naufeæ, 3 coughs, 1 quinfey, 1 fore throat, 1 parotis, 1 with eruptions, 1 fracture of a claviculæ, 2 contufions, 1 wound, 1 fcald, 1 old guinea worm, 1 ulcer, and 1 lame.

Spruce beer was begun to be ferved to the fhip's company on the 17th of the month.

January, 1773.

Notwithftanding this month was much hotter than February laft, when we wereat Sierra Leon the preceding voyage, we had fewer, though a greater variety of patients. The fick lift varied frequently in number, and began to increafe towards the end.

Two remitting fevers occurred, one of which was flight, the other was a healthy young man that had never been in a hot climate before. Though he was

was bad, and continued a confiderable time very weak after his fever, from having a reluctancy to take a proper quantity of bark; there was nothing fingular in his cafe. I prefcribed for him as for the fevers of the former voyage; and in like manner for all the bilious complaints, which foon recovered.

The fore throat and other inflammatory ailments were cured as thofe of January laft, fee page 95 and 96. It is to be obferved that they occurred before the thermometer got high.

The gouty patient was indebted to nature alone for the termination of the fit, by a free perfpiration of the affected part.

They were much afflicted with bilious complaints, and had feveral remitting fevers this month on board of the Difpatch, which moft probably proceeded, in part, from their ufe of the cold bath as often as they had an opportunity after we got to Teneriff. Inftead of its relaxing the pores of their fkins, and thereby promoting a free perfpiration, as they poffibly expected it would do, it naturally produced a contrary effect. They had, in a manner juft left England in the winter feafon, with their fkins, comparatively fpeaking, as dry and tenfe as a piece of parchment, and with ftrong healthful habits; confequently they ftood in no need of a cold bath to brace them more up. I know that in a relaxed habit, when the perfpiration is fuppreffed, or too little in quantity, the cold bath will increafe it by ftrenghing the whole fyftem, but furely their habits were not in that ftate. The cold bath to them who have been a confiderable time in a hot climate, muft, generally fpeaking, be highly beneficial, for obvious reafons; and it is abfolutely neceffary at times, in any climate, for the fake of cleanlinefs, as well as medicinal purpofes: but if people, who are not acquainted with phyfick, go from northern latitudes, in the winter efpecially, to a hot climate, and want to promote a free perfpiration by bathing, immediately upon entering into fuch a climate, they fhould ufe a moderately warm bath, which will foon relax the rigid fibres of the fkin, open the pores thereof, and encreafe the perfpiration. By this method they would obtain their end: however, I am far from being of opinion that it would be a judicious practice, and therefore forbid it.

The beft general preparatives for a change of climate, which I know of, are temperance, and moderate exercife. Evacuations are neceffary in fome habits, efpecially blood letting, but thofe are few compared to the number who do not require them, or may be injured by them.

To return from this digreffion. There were in all added this month to the fick lift, 2 remitting fevers, 3 flight fevers, 4 naufeæ, 1 headach, 1 gout, 1 fore throat, 1 opthalmia, 1 ftrain, 1 contufion, 2 inflammations, 2 abfceffes, 1 guinea worm, and 4 lame patients.

FEBRUARY, 1773.

The people were remarkably healthy notwithſtanding the great number who were employed in wooding and watering the ſhip. None of them ſlept aſhore it is true; but I may, with propriety I think, venture to attribute their entirely eſcaping ſickneſs in thoſe duties, to the tincture of bark having been adminiſtered to every man regularly before they were ſent aſhore in the morning. What principally induced me to make trial of that medicine, as a preventive from fevers, was from recollecting the great benefit which they who ſlept aſhore at the Iſland of St. Thomas, the preceding voyage, found from taking only a ſingle doſe thereof next morning; it, as they themſelves told me, having put new life in them. See the poſtcript, ſection 1.

One half of the few diſeaſes of this month, proceeded from the men's drinking of new fiery ſpirits, which they got from the black people at Cape Coaſt: the belly-ach too, and the nauſeæ of laſt month, moſt probably were owing to their eating plenty of freſh fiſh, unripe plantains, bananas, and what new ſpirits they drank at Sierra Leon, together with the heat of the climate. I preſcribed for them all as in former ſimilar caſes.

The ſick liſt rather decreaſed, all the patients were four ſlight fevers, 2 headachs, 1 belly-ach, 2 rheumatiſms, 1 with eruptions, 1 contuſion, and 1 inflammation.

MARCH, 1773.

The men continued amazingly healthy all this month, if we conſider how great the heat was until the middle thereof; the prodigious quantity of rain which fell, the frequent calms, and the very heavy dews in the nights. Towards the end, the ſick liſt began to encreaſe; there were added to it in all, 2 remitting fevers, 1 ſlight fever, 3 nauſeæ, 1 cold, 1 cough, 1 aſthma, 1 ſore throat, 2 rheumatiſms, 1 nephritis, 1 wound, and 1 lame.

One of the remitting fevers was ſlight, the other was very bad, ſee part iv. § 6. caſe 13. I preſcribed for them as I did for the fevers of the former voyage; and in like manner for all the other patients. One of the nauſeæ was an old man, who was ſpared to a merchant ſhip at Sierra Leon the preceding voyage, but was purpoſely left behind there, by the wretch who commanded her, when he failed. As ſoon as we arrived in the river, he came on board and told his ſtory, and that he had been obliged to the natives for a bare ſubſiſtence. In his countenance both famine and diſeaſe were ſtrongly depicted. I immediately took him under my care; and after a gentle emetick and purge, I gave him four ounces of a wine tincture of bark, twice a day; ſtrictly prohibiting him for a long time from ſalt meat; and interpoſing as I thought fit, both the emetick and the purge. He was afflicted only with very ſlight indiſpoſitions; and was very well when he left us in May, in the Weſt Indies.

The

The ſpruce beer being all expended, wine was begun to be ſerved to the ſhip's company on the 8th of the month. Was ſpruce beer well fermented in hot climates; and if the ſeamen had always moderate labour there; I believe it would be a very ſalutary drink for them. The former was ſeldom the caſe on board the Rainbow, though the latter was during the greateſt part of the time it was ſerved. They who were employed on hard work, cutting the wood, had half a pint of rum, or a pint of wine every man, beſides their beer and tincture of bark every morning.

APRIL, 1773.

There was little alteration in the ſick liſt, before the 15th of the month. The weather then becoming cold, a few feveriſh complaints, ſome rheumatiſms, and ſcorbutic ſymptoms made their appearance; ſo that at the latter end it was conſiderably increaſed. Two of the feveriſh patients became remitting fevers; in one of whom ſigns of the ſcurvy made their appearance, as ſoon as he got over his fever. 2 Remitting fevers, 4 ſlight fevers, 3 headachs, 1 belly-ach, 4 rheumatiſms, 1 opthalmia, and 2 ſcorbutic ulcers, were all the diſeaſes.

With reſpect to the ſcorbutic caſes, I judged wine proper for them, which I did not allow to the other patients. I gave them all the quantity,* with bark and elixir of vitriol; taking care likewiſe to promote the cuticular, and urinary diſcharges, as well as to keep their bodies open with lenitive purges. The ulcers were properly dreſſed too, as often as it ſeemed neceſſary.

Though that method did not cure them, they were much relieved by it. When we arrived at Antigua and St. Kitts, we could neither get fruit, vegetables, nor any freſh proviſions: a violent hurricane which they had had there not long before, having deſtroyed every thing, both in their gardens and fields. I was therefore obliged to perſiſt in my own method with them.

The other patients were treated as ſuch caſes were in former months.

MAY, 1773.

This proved the moſt unhealthy month we had hitherto had, notwithſtanding that very few except ſcorbutic patients were added to the ſick liſt before the 18th, when the dyſentery made its appearance. In all there were added to the ſick liſt, 4 remitting fevers, 1 intermitting fever, 11 ſlight fevers, 4 nauſeæ, 1 headach, 21 dyſenteries, ſome of them mild, 2 diarrhœæ, 9 ſcurvies, 1 with eruptions, 6 contuſions, and 1 lame.

The bilious indiſpoſitions and lame patients were the conſequence of immoderate drinking, and were cured as in former months. The remitting fevers, and

* Here is meant all their allowance, which was a pint daily.

and chiefly all the dyſenteries, I ſent to the hoſpital. Some of the latter recovered on board by evacuations, opiates, and a very light diet. Such were indebted to good conſtitutions, and a favourable attack of the diſeaſe, for their ſpeedy recovery; as it undoubtedly was the ſame diſeaſe with them all. By evacuations here I mean emetics and cathartics only, for not a man was bled. See part IV. § 5. With regard to the method which I followed in the cure, I ſhall briefly inſert it at the end of the review of June.

As this month made ſuch a remarkable change in the health of the people, particularly of the marines, to whom the dyſentery proved to be moſt fatal, it may be worth while to enquire what were the remote, or procatartick, as well as the proximate, or exciting cauſes thereof. An enquiry into theſe cauſes ſeems to be the more neceſſary, becauſe all the other ſhips' companies at Port Royal were healthy; and becauſe there was not a fluxed patient at the hoſpital before our men were ſent to it; where it ſoon ſpread amongſt our ſcorbutic people, from their being together in the ſame wards. I cannot ſuppoſe that there was a particular tendency in the conſtitution of the air, to produce the dyſentery on board of the Rainbow, more than any of the other ſhips which were lying near to us. This enquiry I apprehend, may therefore be made by the following queries—Should they not ſeem to comprehend the real cauſe of the riſe of the flux, as well as of the other diſeaſes? I leave it to every perſon to form his own opinion concerning it.

Though we continued very healthy during the great heat, the very heavy rains, the exceeding denſe and moiſt atmoſphere, and very frequent calms of March; and likewiſe during the month of April, though we had very light winds, and a clouded atmoſphere in the firſt part; and a very cold trade wind in the latter part thereof—Were thoſe circumſtances, together with our long paſſage from Cape Coaſt to Jamaica, upon which the men had neither freſh meat, vegetables, nor fruit, but often in ſhortning ſail, were expoſed to ſcorching heats, deluges of rain, and very cold winds: I ſay, were all thoſe concurring circumſtances ſufficient to form the remote, or procatartick cauſe of the ſcurvy appearing in the end of April; and of the dyſentery in the end of May? Were the immoderate uſe of vegetables, of fruit, of new fiery ſpirits, brackiſh water, which we unfortunately got on board for ſome time, though there is plenty of very good water there, and the very hot weather at Jamaica, ſufficient to form the proximate or exciting cauſe of thoſe diſeaſes, particularly the flux?

By the bye, the ſubject of the former query, that regards the weather, ought to caution others from ever attempting to make their paſſage from the gold coaſt, to any part of the Weſt Indies, or Europe, without going to the ſouthward of the equator. The advantage ariſing from making our paſſage in that manner, the firſt and laſt voyage, appears very evidently in the journal.

With

With refpect to a poffibility to have prevented the dyfentery from being either fo epidemical, or fatal as it was, I beg leave to ftate two more queries.

As the dyfentery did not make its appearance until a week after we arrived at Jamaica—in which time, it was poffible to have got the fhip refitted for fea; and the men could have fupplied themfelves with plenty of vegetables, and fruit; and a fufficient quantity of fugar and coffee, to have ferved them on the paffage to England *—Would it not in all human probability have been prevented from becoming either fo general, or fatal, if we had failed from thence in eight or ten days time?

But as the fhip was detained there fo long, would it not have been the means of repairing, in fome meafure, the injury which the men's health fuftained on the former part of the voyage, to have allowed the fhip's company frefh meat every day, and moft probably of rendering the flux lefs epidemick, and malignant?

However, the Admiral did not think proper to grant either of the applications which were made to him by Captain Collingwood, on both thofe heads.

His Majefty's fhip Phœnix, after having one year made a very long paffage from the coaft of Africa to Jamaica, and being detained there longer than ufual, the men, though they were healthy when the fhip arrived; were feized with a very bad fever, which every one fuppofed would not have happened, had fhe been fent away foon from thence, after her arrival: and that the fever would have proved lefs malignant, if they had been fent home as foon as it made its appearance; and, likewife lefs epidemick. Unlefs therefore his Majefty's fervice abfolutely requires the contrary, the fhip that has been upon the coaft of Guinea, fhould be refitted as fpeedily as poffible, when fhe puts in at Jamaica, and fent home to England.

June, 1773.

The dyfentery ftill continued to rage amongft the people, attacking young and old; but none of the officers was feized with it. However, this is not much to be wondered at, if it is confidered that they lived better in every refpect, and were not near fo much expofed to the many hardfhips which are comprehended in the firft query of the preceding month, as the people were: nor did they afterwards run into the extremes mentioned in the fecond query, as thofe thoughtlefs creatures did.

The attendants of the fick were all taken ill with it. Many of the patients relapfed who were fent from the hofpital as recovered. They who remained on board, efcaped better than them who were at the hofpital; though fome of them alfo relapfed. Four men died of it afhore, and feveral of the nine that came

 on

* Though all feamen are not fo provident as to do fo—many of them are.

on board from thence, very weak. Six of the ten who died in all, were marines.

I cannot help lamenting the fate of the weak hoſpital fluxes, and ſome of the other patients, who ſeemed to ſuffer merely from our anchoring at Blue Field's. They all ſeemingly were recovering; but our ſituation there, as was obſerved in the Journal, page 63, produced an immediate alteration amongſt them for the worſe. The perſpiration being thereby greatly obſtructed, fell conſequently upon the already very weak and relaxed inteſtines, which increaſed the flux; and re-excited the inflammation that ſoon terminated in death by a mortification of the rectum.

The black, putrid, and highly offenſive ſtool or two, which the patient generally voids before death, is an undoubted mark of a mortification's having taken place in the rectum; which they have always found to be the caſe, who have examined the bodies of them who died of the dyſentery. But diſſections not being practiſed on board of his Majeſty's ſhips, unleſs on ſome extraordinary occaſion, I can ſay nothing from my own obſervation of the morbid appearance of the inteſtines of thoſe who died. I ſhall therefore beg leave to refer them who are deſirous of ſuch information, to Sir John Pringle's Obſervations on the Diſeaſes of the Army, page 237; and Cleghorn, on the Diſeaſes of Minorca, page 246. Such an examination of the dead bodies on board of a ſhip, would indeed, not only be attended with much inconvenience; but would likewiſe occaſion much diſcontent, and murmuring amongſt the people, how beneficial ſoever it might afterwards prove to them.

I generally began the cure of the dyſentery, by giving fifteen grains of Ipecacoan in powder; ſometimes, I only gave five or ſix grains, and repeated that quantity two or three times, which was wrought off with warm water. The day after, I ordered an ounce of the common purging ſalts, with manna or coarſe brown ſugar, moſt commonly the latter; or from half a drachm to two ſcruples of rhubarb, ſometimes with nutmeg, and at other times, with two grains of Calomel. The vomit and purge were afterwards repeated as circumſtances required, with an opiate every night from their firſt complaining, and plenty of demulcent drink—either thin water, or rice gruel, barely water, and the white decoction; ſometimes water and a toaſt in it only. When the caſe was favourable, this ſimple method performed the cure.

But when the diſeaſe was violent, and the patients were thereby much reduced in the beginning of their illneſs, as they who came from Port Royal hoſpital were, the flux, violent gripes, with a painful teneſmus, became very obſtinate, and the cure exceedingly difficult. Emollient fomentations for the abdomen, emollient and anticephalick clyſters, beſides internal medicines, and a farinaceous diet, were, I am ſorry to ſay it, too often unſucceſsful. See part IV. chap. II. ſections 5 and 6.

The cure of the remitting fevers, which were not ſent to the hoſpital, and of the bilious complaints, was effected by the method I have already laid down in the former voyage's review. The hæmorrhage was carried off by taking away ſome blood, gentle purges, and a temperate regimen An account of the vomica ſhall be inſerted in next month's review.

All the diſeaſes of June were 24 dyſenteries, 1 diarhœa, 2 remitting fevers, 1 of which was mild, 10 ſlight fevers, 1 cough, 1 vomica, 1 ſore throat, 1 hæmorrhage, 1 ſcurvy, 3 rheumatiſms, 1 muſcular pain of the ſide, 1 ſtrain, 1 contuſion, and 2 lame.

July, 1773.

Though the dyſentery was in its decline, a few very bad caſes happened this month. Two marines died of it: one of whom was at Port Royal hoſpital, the other was added to the ſick liſt in June. He ſeemed to recover until the rainy weather came on, which occaſioned a number of relapſes amongſt the convaleſcent fluxes, but they ſoon recovered. The ſick liſt rather decreaſed all the month, at the end of which, there were only two in it. The patients in all were 16 dyſenteries, many of them mild, 1 diarrhœa, 2 ſlight remitting fevers, 1 cold, 2 rheumatiſms 1 hypochondria, 1 ſcurvy, 1 with eruptions, 1 contuſion, and 1 ulcer I preſcribed for them as in preceding months.

The patient with the vomica, died the 29th of the month. As his caſe appeared ſingular to me, I have inſerted it at length.

The Caſe of the Vomica

Lewis Campbell, ſeaman, aged about 35, rather weakly, had a bad dyſentery, for which he was ſent to Port Royal hoſpital, and returned from thence as cured; but his flux ſoon returned again, and was attended with a ſuppreſſion, and great pain in voiding of his urine. Such medicines as I judged proper, were preſcribed for him. On the fourth day of his relapſe, he complained of a cough, and a pain in his back, beſides of his purging, gripes and teneſmus. As I imagined that the pain of his back proceeded from weakneſs, and his cough from having got a little cold, in turning frequently out of bed in the night to ſtool, I ſtill continued his former medicines. This was on the 17th of June, whilſt we were at Jamaica.

2d Day of his complaining of the cough, he was much the ſame, and his medicines were continued. 3d, He complained of greater pain about his back, and his cough was more urgent and dry. His pulſe was quick and ſmall, and his countenance was fluſhed at times.

I continued

I continued his former medicines, and ordered ten grains of ſperm. cet made into a bolus, with ol. olivar. op. to be taken when the cough was urgent.

4th, He reſted ill in the night. No alteration was made in his medicines, nor on the 5th day. 6th, His flux was better, but his cough was troubleſome. An opiate was preſcribed twice a day, together with his other medicines. 7th, He had a good night. 8th, He complained much of his cough; I repeated his medicines. 9th, He was better and expectorated a very ill concocted matter freely. He was feveriſh at night, as were all the valetudinarian fluxes. I therefore, beſides his former medicines, ordered him the following draught four times a day. ℞ Tinct. cort. vin. ℥i. pulv. cort. peruv. ʒſs. aq. ſimp. ℥iſs. tinct. theb. g. iii. m. 10th, He was much better, though he became feveriſh towards night. His medicines were all repeated. 11th, His flux was abated much, and the teneſmus and gripes were eaſy. He expectorated, particularly in the morning, a large quantity of dark coloured fetid matter, with the cough, after which he found himſelf eaſier. He had been long ſubject to a cough, and complaints in his breaſt, from a hurt which he had formerly received in the right ſide of it—I ordered him a ſoft linctus to uſe often, made of ſperm. cet. mel. Britan. acidulated with ſp. vitr. ten. and a little of the tinct. theb. His drink was a decoction of barley, currants, and liquorice root. 12th, There was no alteration on him. 13th, His flux and its ſymptoms were very moderate; but the expectoration, or rather vomiting of the matter in large quantities every morning, continued, which nearly ſuffocated him. The matter was very offenſive to his taſte and ſmell. Before the vomiting in the morning, the pain of his breaſt, eſpecially of the right ſide, was ſo great, that he could ly on his back only. He had a continual ſmall fever on him; his countenance and hands were ſallow and dirty; his hair was quite dry, and ſtood erect, with a proſtration of his ſtrength and ſpirits. I repeated his medicines, and allowed him a nouriſhing diet. See part iv. end of §. 5.

14th, He was much the ſame, and complained more of his flux and gripes. His medicines were continued. The fit of vomiting the matter commonly happened in the morning with his cough, when he was at ſtool, which perhaps, was owing to all the matter diſcharged from the ulcer in the night, either falling down, or bearing upon the diaphragma.

15th, He had a very reſtleſs night with his cough. I ordered his medicines to be repeated. P. m. he was frequently purged and griped in the day. 16th, There was no alteration for the better. He took his medicines regularly. 17th, He was very weak from the flux, cough, and vomiting of the fetid pus, which was highly offenſive to him, He now likewiſe expectorated a great quantity throughout the day and night. I continued his linctus, ptiſan, opiates and diet,

diet, allowed him half a pint of wine,* and gave him an ounce of the tinct cort. vin. four times a day. 18th, No alteration appeared on him.

19th, He expectorated the pus in greater quantities through the day with his cough, of the ſame dark colour. The hectick fever, and the fluſhing of his countenance continued with partial colliquative ſweats. He had very little appetite, and was thirſty in the nigh I omitted the linctus, and again rdered him the bark as on the 9th, and continued his ptiſan, opiates, wine, and diet.

20th, He was no better, and was extremely weak, and his countenance was much fallen. I preſcribed five doſes of the bark. 21ſt, He had a better night than uſual, and he was more chearful. I ordered him ſix doſes of the bark. His opiate was now a grain and a half of opium. 22d, He reſted worſe than in the preceding night. He expectorated and puked a quart of pus in twenty-four hours---his flux and gripes were very moderate. I increaſed the doſe to two ſcruples of the bark, and gave him ſix doſes in the day, with his drink, diet, wine and opiates as before.

23d, He was reſtleſs in the night, and very feveriſh. I repeated all his medicines. 24th, There was little or no alteration. 25th, He reſted much better in the night, his flux was gone, and he expectorated leſs: he was ſick at the ſtomach; I ordered him ten grains of ipecacoan, which puked him, and gave him two copious ſtools. During the time of his vomiting his noſe bled a little. Afterwards, he took his bark and wine as before. 26th, He was in much better ſpirits, and he looked better. I repeated his bark, with his other medicines and diet as before.

27th, He had now ſeldom the hectick heats, colliquative ſweats or thirſt, and was regaining both his appetite and ſtrength. He coughed little, expectorated moderately, the pus was no longer fetid or offenſive to his taſte, and was of a laudable colour and conſiſtence. He told me that the flies and inſects which, before he began to take the bark, always devoured the pus, would not touch it now. The attendants and people about him made the ſame obſervation: I gave ſix drachms of the bark in the day, in the ſame manner as before; he only took an opiate at night.

28th, He found himſelf much better, and complained of no pain about his breaſt, but when he lay on his right ſide. p. m. By the wine being omitted with his bark, without my knowledge, he puked and had ſeveral ſtools, and was feveriſh at night. 29th, He reſted very indifferently in the night, and had little appetite. I ordered his medicines, wine, and diet to be repeated. His opiate for ſome nights paſt, was two grains of the opium. 30th, He was much better, his medicines and diet agreeing with him. p. m. The

cough,

* It is to be obſerved that the meaſures in the navy are one eighth leſs than they are aſhore.

cough, the pain of his breaſt, and hectick fever returned. 31ſt, He was very indifferent, after a reſtleſs night. I order'd him two ſcruples of rhubarb, and only half an ounce of bark at four doſes, with wine, and his opiate. The rhubarb gave him two copious ſtools.

32d, He was much better after a tolerable night's reſt. He took his bark. 33d, He continued better, and perſpired freely. I repeated his bark, wine, and opiate. 34th, He complained of weakneſs only, expectorated a little laudable pus, and had no bad ſymptoms about him. I continued his medicines. 35th, He had ſeveral ſtools in the night. I preſcribed his medicines and diet as before. 36th, His perſpiration ſtopt, he was griped and frequently purged in the night. Moſt probably from the diſagreeable change of weather. See the journal page 66. I preſcribed a doſe of rhubarb, and afterwards his bark, wine, and opiate as before. 37th, He paſſed a reſtleſs night from the grips and his fever. a. m. He complained leſs tho' he was very feveriſh. I repeated his bark and wine. p. m. He was hot, thirſty, very much dejected, and complained of great weakneſs. I gave him his opiate.

38th, His flux continued, he had a ſhort, dry, urgent cough, and he was much weaker and deſponding. I omitted the bark, and preſcribed the diaſcord mixture with his wine and ſmall doſes of opium. p. m. He was more feveriſh and began to rave. 39th, He was much worſe; his pulſe was very ſmall and quick, he was very thirſty, and raved more, and was hungry. I repeated his medicines as on the 38th day. p. m. His extremities became cold, he was quite reſtleſs, and his pulſe was very irregular, and ſeemed to vibrate at times. I order'd him wine only. 40th, He had one ſtool in the night. His countenance was *hippocratick*; there was a cadaverous ſmell about him, and he grew much weaker. I continued his wine. 41ſt, His countenance was frequently diſtorted with convulſive twitches; he muttered deliriouſly, and was quite reſtleſs with his limbs. His pulſe was thready and tremulous, and his hands were convulſed. In this manner he died at midnight.

Had we been ſo fortunate as to have had good weather a fortnight, or three weeks longer, until he had recover'd more ſtrength, in all probability he would have got well.

August, 1773.

It being rainy until the 20th of the month, the 7th and 12th days excepted, the ſick liſt continued encreaſing. 11 Dyſenteries, chiefly relapſes; 1 headach; 1 cough; 1 ſcurvy; 1 rheumatiſm; 3 contuſions; 1 opthalmia; 1 abſceſs; and 1 with a dimneſs of ſight, in all, complained.

One of the relapſed dyſenteries died, who was highly ſcorbutick, and a conſiderable time bad before he complained. See caſe VI. of the Jamacia dyſentry.

A marine

A marine likewife died of it: a very bad fever attended his flux. See the cafe preceding the one juft referred to.

All the patients were treated as in former fimilar cafes.

Ten of the men died this voyage of the dyfentery. Four died at Port Royal hofpital, and fix on the paffage from Jamaica to England; four of whom had been at the hofpital. I reckon the patient who had the vomica one of the four. One man fell over board and was drowned on the paffage from Jamaica.

CHAPTER III.

Review of the Sick List, with Practical Observations from the 21ft of November 1773, to the 1ft of September, 1774.

November and December, 1773.

THE people continued amazingly healthy during the time that the fhip ftayed in England, confidering their irregularities and indifcretion. One man was drowned along fide of the hulk, which the men were on board of, whilft the fhip was in dock; 1 was killed by a fall from the fhip's fide into the dock; 6 weak from fluxes and other difeafes; 6 fevers; 4 with the rheumatifm; 2 fluxes; 2 coughs; 1 ulcer; and 1 contufion, were fent to the hofpital in that time, befides thofe men who were fent the day after our arrival from Jamaica.

The patients who were in the fick lift when we failed, proceeded, as thofe in the former voyages, from great intemperance and then getting cold; and their number continued to encreafe until the end of December, when it was the fame as at the time of our leaving England.

A new fever appeared on board the 13th of December, whilft we lay at Teneriff. I call it a new one becaufe it did not occur in any of the other two preceding voyages: an account of which I fhall infert at the end of next month's review, and call it a catarrhous fever.

All the difeafes of the month were 3 remitting fevers, which were mild, 6 flight fevers, 7 catarrhous fevers, 1 intermitting fever, 1 diarrhœa, 1 cough, 1 fcurvy, 2 rheumatifms, 1 hamorrhoides, 1 with eruptions, 1 weak, 1 nephrites, 5 contufions, 1 ftrain, 2 inflammations, 1 abfcefs, and 3 ulcers.

I prefcribed

I prefcribed for the feverifh indifpofitions as already mentioned, page 74, and for the chirurgical patients, after the manner I have fet down for contufions, page 96, excepting the abfcefs and ulcers. The laft of which will be fpoken of hereafter. Concerning an abfcefs I need fay nothing. The hemorrhoids were cured by keeping the body open with a common purging electury, to which flos. fulph. was added, after giving a fmart purge, by the ufe of a fomentation, and anointing the parts with an emollient ointment, containing fulphur.

The fcurvy appeared in the patient's ankle a few days after we failed. The caufe of which proceeded moft probably, from his having been put in irons when drunk a little time before, when it was ftrained. He foon became exceedingly bad, being fcarce able to ftand with the help of crutches. I ordered him lime juice with wine and fugar twice a day, and a proper regimen, fee part IV. ch. 1. § 5. which recovered him in a great meafure, but he did not get quite well on board.

January, 1774.

The fick lift varied little, though it rather decreafed all the month. In the beginning thereof a few catarrhous fevers were added to it, and were fucceeded by bilious complaints. The patients in all were 3 remitting fevers, 1 of them only was bad, 7 flight fevers, 4 catarrhous fevers, 1 belly-ach, 1 contufion 1 inflammation, and 2 lame. I prefcribed for the bilious complaints as in February 1772.

The Catarrhous Fever defcribed.

The catarrhous fever attacked both young and old, and it was remarkable, that a few who were firft taken ill with it, and towards its declenfion likewife, had it in a more favourable manner than the intermediate number. What were either the procatartick, or the proximate caufes thereof, I know not perfectly. I have mentioned in the journal, fee the 23 of February 1772, that the Weafel's men were feized with catarrhous complaints whilft they lay off Senegal, in very foggy weather, which probably occafioned them: but in the Rainbow, the fever commenced at Teneriff, and difappeared whilft we lay off Senegal, in very indifferent weather, as is evident from the journal.

In fome patients this fever began with a fwelling, and pain in one fide of the face, and throat; but generaly the whole face and throat was fwelled, the feat of which fwelling feemed to be in the glands, though they were not remarkably hard. The uvula, tonfils, and fublingual glands were enlarged and redder than natural. The fwelling was painful, the patient was feverifh, and at night there was an exacerbation. About the third day, the fwelling was much

much increafed, the whole head being affected. They fpoke with pain, deglutition was difficult, and the fever with thirft, was more confiderable. The fixth day, the fwelling, pain and fever were much abated; but they ftill had pain in fwallowing. They complained of an offenfive tafte and fmell in their mouths and throats, although I never perceived an abfcefs, or an ulcer in them.

Moft of them recovered in eight days; a few fooner; one recovered on the 11th, and one was afterwards feifed with a cough and a very bad fever. See cafe 15th of the fever, part IV.

The crifis was a free perfpiration about the throat, and a copious falivation, attended with the offenfive tafte and fmell already mentioned.

From the general part of them, I took away a little blood, which was fomewhat fizy, and next day ordered a purge of falts, which I repeated as occafion required, efpecially when the bad tafte and fmell was perceived. I afterwards gave the faline mixture with Huxham's effence of antimony, from fifteen to forty drops, every fix hours; allowed them fage tea or barley water for drink; made them gargle frequently, with decoct. falv. mel. Britan. & acet. diftil. embrocated externally with the volatile liniment, and covered the parts with flannel; and prefcribed a light diet.

February, 1774.

The patients were not numerous this month, and were chiefly bilious indifpofitions; moft probably they proceeded from their eating unripe plantains, bananas, plenty of frefh fifh, and the hot weather. I ordered fuch medicines for them as I have already mentioned. See page 97.

Two remitting fevers occurred, one of which was mild---this man had been in the fick lift not long before, with a bilious complaint---the other was mortal.

Though I have faid he died of a remitting fever, ftrictly fpeaking, it had neither the pathognomonick fymptoms of the fever, nor of the dyfentery, as may be feen from his cafe in the following month's review, and may therefore be more properly called *anomalous*.

The fick lift decreafed until the 10th of the month, and then increafed until the end. All the difeafes were 2 remitting fevers, 6 flight fevers, 4 diarrhœæ, 1 belly-ach, 1 cough, 1 hypochondria, 1 with piles, 2 with eruptions, 1 fcrophula, 1 ftrain, 2 contufions, 1 ulcer, and 1 lame.

March, 1774.

The fhip's company was remarkably healthy all the month, which I may again venture to fay, was principally owing to the tincture of bark having been adminiftered to all the people who were employed on fhore duty, after the fame

 manner

manner as it was the preceding voyage. This circumſtance deſerves the more particular attention, becauſe they had not the advantage of getting any freſh ſtock, when the ſhip was at the Cape de Verde iſlands, as they had the two preceding voyages. Another circumſtance is worthy of notice—the marine who got drunk, and lay in the woods one night, and amongſt the blacks the following night, at Sierra Leon, when ſent as one of the wooding party, as I have remarked in the journal, page 76, 77, and 78, never had the leaſt ailment, from my having taken the precaution of giving him the bark, after a vomit and purge.

The ſick liſt continued to decreaſe until the 24th of the month, when a few ſlight ailments were added to it. The opthalmia remitted, and after vomiting and purging the patient, it was carried off by the bark. The old ſcorbutick patient recovered amazingly, from being ſent aſhore at Sierra Leon, and Cape Coaſt every day, though he was a dirty inclined wretch. The hypochondria grew worſe, and he was ſo obſtinate who had it, that he would take no medicines. I preſcribed for the other diſeaſes as in preceding months. The man with the fiſtula in ano, had only a ſmall draining from a part of the old inciſion, where he had formerly been cut for a fiſtula. His body was kept open, and dreſſings applied to the part.

In all were added to the ſick liſt, 4 ſlight fevers; 1 darrhœa, 1 opthalmia, and a few ſlight complaints of the ſame kind; 1 excoriation, and 1 old fiſtula in ano. The anomalous caſe of laſt month, died the 6th of this: and now follows

The Anomalous Caſe.

Wm. Macartney, ſeaman, aged about fifty-ſix years, after having been a month bad, complained on the 24th of February, while we lay at Sierra Leon, of a purging with ſevere gripes, of a puking, a headach, thirſt, great weakneſs, and univerſal pains. His countenance was ſallow, and he had very little fever. I ordered fifteen grains of ipecacoan, and an opiate at bed time, with barley water for his drink.

2d Day of his complaining, there was no alteration: I preſcribed two ſcruples of rhubarb. *p. m.* He was griped all the day, and had only one ſtool. An emollient clyſter was therefore adminiſtered, and his opium—half a grain, repeated at night.

3d, He had a bad night; the gripes were conſtant, with a fruitleſs deſire of going to ſto l. I ordered pulv. ipecacoan. gr. v. tinct. theb. gt. vi. aq. ſimp. ℥iſs. ſyr. ſim. ʒii. fiat hauſtus ter in die ſumendus. *p. m.* He found himſelf rather eaſier, and his thirſt leſs, but his medicine had puked him only. The clyſter

clyſter was therefore repeated, and his anodyne at night. I allowed him a little wine

4th, He paſſed a reſtleſs night, and was not relieved by his clyſter, though it gave him ſeveral copious ſtools: I repeated his doſe of rhubarb and anodyne, with his wine. *p. m.* He had ſeveral ſtools; he was very weak, his ſpirits were much depreſſed, he had no appetite, and his gripes continued with a ſmall fever upon him.

5th, He found himſelf no better. He had been long ſubject to complaints in his bowels, from the dry belly-ach, which he had formerly had in the Weſt Indies. *a. m.* I ordered him two of the following pills, with plenty of demulcent drink, (ſee page 108) and his opiate at night. ℞. pulv. r. rhei ʒi. tart. emet. gr. iv. ſapon. ven. gr. viii. tinct. thebaic. gt. xxxvi. ſyr. ſimp. fiat maſſa pilularum dividenda in No. xii *a. m.* He had no ſtool: the clyſter was repeated.

6th, He reſted a little better; his clyſter procured him but one ſtool. The abdomen was ſwelled and tenſe, and the ſmall fever ſtill continued: I repeated the pills, and ordered the abdomen to be well fomented, which gave him eaſe. *p. m.* His countenance was gaſtly. I preſcribed camphor gr. vi and gave him his wine and opiate.

7th, He paſſed a bad night; he dozed with his eyes half open, and was in no reſpect better, though he had two copious ſtools in the night. *p. m.* He was no eaſier. I repeated his pills, and gave him ten grains of camphor, with his anodyne and wine. 8th, He had ſeveral ſtools in the night; nevertheleſs, the ſwelling, and tenſion of the abdomen was very troubleſome. I ordered his medicines, wine, and drink to be continued. *p. m.* His body was lax.

9th, The abdomen was more diſtended and hard, though not conſtipated, nor had he any obſtruction of his urine. His pulſe was very ſmall, his ſkin was only moderately warm, and his thirſt nevertheleſs, was inſatiable. I again preſcribed as before. 10th, He had a very reſtleſs night: the abdomen was painful upon being touched; and he was ſeized with bilious vomitings, and a hiccup. *p. m.* As he had only one ſtool, I ordered the clyſter to be repeated, and his medicines and wine to be continued. 11th, He was extremely reſtleſs in the night, and the ſwelling and tenſion of the abdomen increaſed. I preſcribed wine only. *p. m.* He had two copious ſtools in no wiſe putrid, and died at four o'clock.

April, 1774.

The firſt day of the month, a very malignant dyſentery made its appearance amongſt the marines, who were the greateſt ſufferers therein, as well as in the dyſentery of the preceding voyage Several of the ſeamen were attacked with the ſcurvy; a few with bilious indiſpoſitions; and two with remitting fevers, of of which one was of a mild form. In all 13 dyſenteries, 1 diarrhœa, 2 belly-achs, 2 remitting fevers, 2 nauſeæ, 1 headach, 4 ſcurvies, 1 rheumatiſm, and 1 excoriation, were added to the ſick liſt. As we may therefore juſtly be ſaid to have had a very quick tranſition from a healthy to a ſickly ſtate, I beg leave to ſtate the following queries concerning it, and ſhall leave it to every perſon to judge whether or not they expreſs the real cauſes of the tranſition.

Could our long inactive ſituation off Senegal Bar, without freſh meat, and vegetables, in a very impure atmoſphere, (ſee the Journal, page 73 and 74) the diſappointment of our not getting any freſh ſtock at the Cape de Verde iſlands immediately after; and the men's remarkable great abuſe of new ſpirits while the ſhip lay at Cape Coaſt, be ſaid to be the remote or procatartick cauſes of the ſickly change?

Could the two rainy laſt days of March be ſaid to have been the proximate or immediate exciting cauſe of it?

It is true that a boat came on board of us twice, on the 31ſt of March, from the whale fiſhing veſſel, and brought the maſter of her, who was bad of a Tertian fever of a mild form; but as all the reſt of her men were well, it can hardly be ſuppoſed that a dyſenterick infection was contracted from him; beſides the marine who firſt complained of the dyſentery, was taken ill the 3 ſt of March. Allowing then that a malignant dyſentry could have been originated from a mild remitting fever, which is by no means probable, is it to be ſuppoſed, that the infection would have operated ſo powerfully as to have produced its fatal effect (I may ſay) inſtantaneouſly?

The preceding voyage indeed, we had no flux on the paſſage from the coaſt of Africa to Jamaica, notwithſtanding all the heavy rains: but there were not the previous concurring circumſtances to them, which we met with the laſt voyage. The men too no doubt got drunk the former voyages, when the ſhip was at Cape Coaſt, at times; but they were hardly ever ſober while we lay there the laſt voyage.

Whether there was any particular diſpoſition in the conſtitution of the air to introduce the dyſentery immediately with the rains laſt voyage, or not, I will not preſume to ſay, nor offer any hypotheſis on the ſubject. I have ſtated all the facts which were obvious, concerning it, that every perſon may form his own judgment of the matter; for I acknowledge myſelf to be no admirer of hypotheſes in the practice of phyſick, be they ever ſo ſpecious. They may indeed ſhow the ingenuity of the authors, but, in my opinion, they never can be really ſerviceable.

The dyſentery of which we are now ſpeaking, run more ſpeedily through its different ſtages, than that which occurred the preceding voyage; conſequently it was more ſpeedily fatal. Three marines and the ſhip's barber died: not an officer,

officer, or petty officer was ſeized with it Probably, for the very ſame reaſons which I alledged for their having eſcaped it the preceding voyage.

For a particular account of it, and of the manner in which I preſcribed for it, ſee the general account of the dyſentery, part IV. ch. 2. I preſcribed for all the other diſeaſes as in ſuch caſes of former months.

May, 1774.

Five ſick people were left at Antigua hoſpital. The ſick liſt increaſed all the month, of which the diſeaſes were various, though not a dyſenterick patient complained before the 15th Day, after which a few very bad caſes thereof were added to the ſick liſt. Moſt of them were ſent to Port Royal hoſpital, where it attacked our own ſcorbutic men, from the ſame cauſe that it did the preceding voyage.

The ſcurvey continued to prevail amongſt the ſeamen until we arrived at Port Royal. However, they were not numerous even then, nor were any of them bad, except the patients who had ulcers, which became very foul, and troubleſome.

The remitting fevers were chiefly mild; but a few of the patients were liable to relapſes, as was one man with a headach which remitted, and he continued long weak. The bilious complaints were moſtly added about the end of the month, after the people had got new rum.

All the diſeaſes of the month were 8 remitting fevers, chiefly mild; 2 ſlight fevers, 3 headachs, 8 dyſenteries, 1 diarrhæa, 1 belly-ach, 6 ſcurvies, 1 cough, 1 mortification, with eruptions, 1 ſcald, 1 contuſion, 1 lame, and 4 ſcorbutick ulcers.

In preceding months, I have mentioned in what manner I preſcribed for ſimilar caſes—excepting the mortification; but I ſhall here add ſome remarks concerning the ſcurvy, and then relate the caſe of the mortification at length.

Some Remarks on the Scurvy.

Amongſt the ſcorbutick patients during the ſecond and laſt voyage, for there were none the firſt: no unuſual ſymptoms appeared, that is to ſay, no other ſymptom than is already taken notice of by the indefatigable Doctor Lind, in his moſt elaborare treatiſe on that diſeaſe. It would therefore be needleſs for me to enumerate their general complaints, or to inſert any particular caſe, as nothing, I believe, can be added to his complete hiſtory of it, or to the method which he has laid down for curing it, in the third edition of his book.

All that I ſhall therefore add on this head, is, that the ſcorbutick people on board the Rainbow, were treated whilſt ſhe was at ſea, as nearly as circumſtances would admit, after the judicious method which Dr. Lind has laid down; but none of them were perfectly recovered when we arrived at Jamaica, where they were all ſent aſhore to Port Royal hoſpital, and had a freſh meat diet, with plenty of vegetables and fruit.

The laſt voyage however, I ſelected three patients whoſe caſes were nearly ſimilar, to make an experiment with different medicines. The three were upon the ſame regimen, and had each of them a pint of wine daily. To the patient who was oldeſt, and rather the worſt, I gave twice a day, one ounce of lime juice, and two ounces of wine mixed and ſweetned with coarſe brown ſugar; to the youngeſt of the three, I gave the elixir of vitriol twice a day in water, in ſuch a quantity, as not to gripe him; and for the other patient who was elderly, and the ſecond in illneſs, I ordered an ounce of the bark in powder every day, mixed with water only.

The medicines were regularly adminiſtered for a week, at the end of which it was evident that the man who had taken the bark was by much the moſt relieved, for he then complained only of weakneſs, he found himſelf ſo much recovered. Next to him, the old man who had taken the lime juice mixture, was the moſt relieved. But I could obſerve no alteration for the better in his caſe who took the elixir of vitriol.

Before I quit this ſubject, I muſt beg leave to add one remark, which may not be altogether unworthy of the attention of ſome of my brethren. It is certain, that a few caſes of any particular diſeaſe, can ſeldom preſent to a phyſician or ſurgeon, all the variety of ſymptoms, which are contained in the general hiſtory thereof; becauſe a general hiſtory is, undoubtedly, compiled from a greater number of caſes, than can poſſibly fall under the obſervation of every practitioner. Therefore, though the pathognomonick ſymptoms will generally indicate to an old practitioner the real diſeaſe; yet it is more than probable, when a few caſes only happen to fall under the care of a younger, which do not preſent all the various ſymptoms that are ſet forth in the general hiſtory of that diſeaſe, and which they are only acquainted with from reading, that this is the principal cauſe of their being puzzled in diſtinguiſhing the diſeaſe, and in treating ſuch patients properly.

I only ſay, that the pathognomonick ſymptoms will generally indicate what diſeaſe it is, becauſe ſometimes, the caſe is ſo complex, as to baffle all the ſkill of the moſt diſcerning phyſician to inveſtigate. When that occurs, all that can poſſibly be done, I apprehend, is to ſubdue the moſt alarming ſymptoms one after another, until the diſeaſe is either perfectly cured, or aſſumes its proper type.

What led me to this reflection, was my recollecting a ſcorbutick patient's caſe

case which occurred to me on board of his Majesty's sloop Ferret, in the bay of Mexico, in the year 1766. On a very short cruise from Pensacola, (after the ship's company had been a long time without fresh meat or vegetables,) in that bay, we had extremely bad weather, during which the people were often wet and greatly fatigued. The scurvy soon made its appearance, attacked a number, and was very rapid in its progress.

Having unfortunately lost my day-book, I cannot mention all the particulars relating to the man's case, but I remember well, that it corresponded very nigh with the uncommon appearance (of an universal dropsy) which it put on in the East Indies, on board of his Majesty's squadron in the late war, as described in Doctor Lind's treatise; † which appearance I had not heard of then, far less seen, though I had an opportunity of seeing the scurvy in all its stages, on board of his Majesty's ship Prince of Orange, on a cruise in the bay, after the reduction of Belle Isle, when we had above a hundred men bad, of whom, fortunately, only one died. I was therefore so much puzzled, that I consulted Doctor Lorimer * at Pensacola on his case, and by his advice I made different times several punctures with a lancet in the scrotum, which was greatly distended, as well as his whole body, when the disease was in an advanced state, and treated him in every respect as if his disease had been an anasarcha; but he died soon after I left the Ferret. So that Doctor Lorimer did not suspect his case to be scorbutick, more than I did then.

None of the Ferret's men died except that poor man, although several of them were in the last stage of the disease before they were got ashore. But they were certainly indebted for their recovery, to the humany of Governor Johnston, and Captain Murray who commanded her. The one generously spared his country house for an hospital, and gave them fresh salad every day: and the other allowed them his wine in such quantities as I thought proper.

The Case of the Gangrene or Mortification.

Charles Duplassey, butcher, an old man, much given to drinking, was subject to the gout, and gravelish complaints with a suppression of his urine; the last of which generally followed his being drunk, and was carried off by gentle cathartics, diureticks, and a pediluvium. On the evening of the 9th of May, he complained of being unable to make water, and of great pain about the penis. Upon examination, I found both the penis and scrotum much enlarged, and of an inflated appearance, which I supposed was the consequence of the urine's

† See page 278, of the third edition.

* This gentleman is yet Surgeon General of the province of West Florida, and remarkable for his knowledge of mathematicks, as well as eminent in his profession.

urine's having been fuppreffed fome time, as he upon my enquiring acknowleged had been the cafe, I ordered him a ftrong decoction of rad. alth. and fal nitr. with fugar, to be drank frequently; the parts to be ftuped with a difcutient fomentation, and to be fufpended; and made him ufe a pediluvium. His medicine operated by ftool and urine, but not freely.

Next evening he complained of flatulencies in his bowels, and a flight reaching at times. The inflated-like tumour did not fubfide, nor was his pain leffened. I was aftonifhed the morning of the 11th to fee the fcrotum in a ftate of mortification. He complained too of much pain about the pubis, which gradually afcended to the abdomen; all the pubis was fomewhat red; the fpermatick cords were much enlarged, tenfe, and exceedingly painful, as were the penis and fcrotum, upon being ever fo gently handled. His pulfe was languid, and he had frequent cold clamy fweats on him. I added fpirit of wine to the fomentation and dreffed the parts with hot digeftives. I ordered him the bark in equal parts of red port and water as often as his ftomach would receive it. He took to the quantity of a drachm and a half of the bark every hour at leaft, with thirty drops of the fp. nitr. dulc. at times; but towards night the mortification had feized the prepuce which was very large, and the penis was become emphyfematous. He made water in a fmall quantity, and had no appetite from his firft complaining;— he was now troubled with a hiccup; and his pulfe was very weak and irregular. In the morning of the 12th his extremities became cold, there was a cold clammy fweat on him; he was now infenfible; his breathing was laborious; and his pulfe was thready and fluttered before he died at 9 a.m. The mortification externally, did not penetrate deeper than the fkin. The fœtor about him even before his death, was exceffively offenfive.

After he died, I was informed * that he was very drunk the afternoon of the 7th, and lay with a black woman that night, who had *blown* him; and hat he was taken ill the next morning, though he did not complain—the pain and fwelling about the genitals having begun then. What was meant by his having been *blown* by the woman, I was ignorant of; but hearing at the fame time, that there was a man in the fhip who had formerly fuftained a like injury from a whore, I fent for him to afk him fome queftions on the fubject. " He told me that he faw the butcher's condition the morning after he lay with the black whore, and then mentioned to him what the matter was with him; that he likewife had been ferved fo by a girl, and was fent to an hofpital, where he was all cut and recovered; but that he told the furgeon thereof by what means it happened." He was a young healthy man. " He added that the whore meth

* I have no great faith in the following relation, which is inferted in the manner that I had it; only becaufe I thought it curious.

method of ſerving him the trick, he could not tell, for he perceived no unuſual circumſtance in the act of coition that ſhe did. However, added he, he was certain that ſhe knew of her having done it, becauſe ſhe ran away as ſoon as ſhe got out of bed, and never went near him again; and he ſuppoſed that ſhe had ſerved him ſo for beating her before they went to bed. He further added, that the butcher had beat his girl before they went to bed, and ſhe likewiſe went aſhore as ſoon as ſhe got up in the morning, and never returned to him."

From the preceding relation (which I learned too late, to make any experiment in the butcher's caſe; and if I had known it ſooner, I am doubtful whether I could have been the means of preſerving his life, by reaſon of his age, bad conſtitution, and his being ſo long in complaining after he found himſelf bad) it would appear, that only ſome proſtitutes have this infernal art of *blowing* a man in the act of coition. My mate, who had ſeen numbers of ſuch caſes, never once ſuſpected it to be the butcher's, nor mentioned it until I told him what the young man ſaid, but he could give me no information that was ſatisfactory about the matter; neither could ſome eminent Phyſicians whom I have ſince conſulted thereon, notwithſtanding they had had ſome caſes of the ſame kind under their care in their courſe of practice. As for my own part, I ſtill confeſs myſelf perfectly ignorant of it; but if it really is in the power of a proſtitute to commit ſo helliſh a trick, I think it very providential that ſo few of them know the art, otherwiſe I may venture to ſay, that they would treat men in that abominable manner for every ſlight offence.

Query. May the people's drinking new rum at Antigua and St. Kitts; the heavy rains of the 19th and 20th of the Month, to which all of them were expoſed; and their great abuſe of new rum, vegetables and fruit, immediately after at Jamaica; be ſaid to be the exciting cauſes of the Dyſentery re-appearing again, as well as of the bilious complaints?

And may not the ſame queries be ſtated here, as were laſt May, reſpecting the poſſibility of either preventing the dyſentery from becoming ſo epidemick, or rendering it leſs malignant?---Some of the men died of it at the Hoſpital.

June, 1774.

The patients were very few this Month, and their complaints were the evident effects of their intemperance, and indiſcretion. Four were added to the ſick liſt the firſt day; from that until the middle, one now and then only; after which they were more frequent. None of them were dangerouſly ill except the patient with the remitting fever, who got bad from fatigue and expoſing himſelf too much to the ſun: He was ſent to ſick quarters the third day of his illneſs: ſee the laſt caſe of the remitting fever, Part IV. Moſt of the other patients were ſent to the hoſpital. The few who remained on board were treated as ſuch diſeaſes in ſo mer Months. In all they were 3 Dyſenteries; 1 Diarrhæa; 1 remitting Fever; 3 flight Fevers; 1 Headach; 1 Scurvy; 1 Hectick patient; 1 Contufion; 1 Lame; 1 Wound, and 1 Ulcer.

The patient with the fcurvy was the Marine, who was fo dangeroufly ill after the catarrhous fever; and the only marine who had the fcurvy in the three voyages.

The patients of this Month were ftill fewer than thofe of the laft, unlefs we include them who returned from the Hofpital, and were added to the fick lift, and the feven invalids. They who came from the Hofpital were 4 fcorbutick fluxes; 1 epilepfy, who was fent for a dyfentary; 1 dyfentary; 1 valetudinarian flux; 1 fcrophula; and 1 contufion. The invalids were 1 blind of an eye; 1 gout; 1 with obftructions in the abdomen from a remitting fever; 1 headach from an old fracture of the cranium; 1 very large foul ulcer; and 2 chronic fluxes; moft of whom recovered much, from the medicines which I had hitherto prefcribed in fimilar cafes.

One of the fcorbutick fluxes that returned from the hofpital, was feized on the 20th with a flow nervous fever, which cafe fhall be defcribed at the end of the review of Auguft.---The contufion I difcovered to be a fracture of the head of the os femoris but I could then be of no real fervice, it happening when I was a fhore, and my mate, before he fent him, nor the furgeons at the hofpital, never fufpected it. Epithems and a regimen were all that I could prefcribe for him. The fcrophulous arm was laid open at the hofpital, and was now exceffively troublefome and painful to the poor man, who was greatly reduced by the dyfentery, which attacked him there, and continued to hang upon him, in fpite of every method that I could think of to remove it. Applications were of very little benefit to the arm.---The epilepfy continued as obftinate as it had been at the hofpital, where he got it by a fright one night in bed, he faid. Evacuations, blifters, gum pills, volatiles, opiates, bark and the cold bath, were not fuccefsful, in the manner they were tried afhore, and all repeated again on board. The fit always occurred in the night, and at times he efcaped having a fit for one night, or fometimes had a flight one; but thefe circumftances were uncertain, and feldom. As I did not fee him until he had been bad a confiderable time, I think it would be needlefs to infert only a part of his cafe.

There was nothing particular in any of the difeafes which were added on board---namely, 4 flight fevers; 1 head ach, 1 naufea; 2 belly-achs; 1 flow nervous fever; 1 epilepfy; 1 contufion; 1 fracture—difcover'd; and 2 lame patients. The old hypochondriac patient continued very obftinate, and would take no medicine.

AUGUST,

August, 1774.

The weather being rainy, the ſick liſt increaſed until the 26th of the month and afterwards decreaſed. As we were daily raiſing our latitude, at the ſame time it became colder, eſpecially at the latter end of the month; the diſeaſes therefore chiefly aroſe from that cauſe, many of the people being ill provided for ſuch a change of weather, which is generally the caſe with them after leaving a hot climate, as I have already obſerved. However, they were not numerous, the phyſical patients were all relapſes, and one of the intermittents was an invalid; ſome of rheumatiſms were relapſes, and the reſt who had it were ſubject to it---except the complaints which were added the two laſt days; there were but few in the liſt when we arrived in England, unleſs we include the invalids who were all amazingly recovered; but him with the blind eye, the man with the large foul ulcer, and him with the obſtructions of the abdomen were quite well; the laſt of whom was recovered by purges of jalap and calomel, frequently repeated, and in the intervals pills of ſoap and emetick tartar, and a light diet with wine.

All that were added to the ſick liſt were, 1 remitting fever; 3 intermitting fevers; 1 of whom was an invalid; 1 ſlight fever; 1 head ach; 1 belly ach; 5 rheumatiſms; 4 contuſions; 1 ſcald; and 1 wound.

I preſcribed for them as I had done for ſimilar caſes hitherto.

The man with the ſlow nervous fever of laſt month, was returned to his duty the 14th of this, quite well, whoſe caſe I ſhall now inſert.

The Caſe of the ſlow Nervous Fever.

Charles Burton, ſeaman, aged about 28, of a effeminate temper, complained on the 10th of May ult. of ſcorbutick ſymptoms, for which he was ſent to Port Ro al hoſpital the 22d, and continued there until we ſailed from Jamaica, where he had a ſlight attack of the dyſentery. A conſiderable time after he came on board he was feeble, and was troubled with a cough, notwithſtanding he took medicines and was under a proper regimen. He complained the 19th of July that he had had a purging on him for three days, altho' he did not mention it, for which I ordered him then three doſes of ipecacoan, each five grains, and an anodyne at night.

On the 20th of July, latitude obſerved at noon 18° 58 N. though his purging was abated, he complained of unuſual weakneſs, heat, and thirſt. P. M. he was very peeviſh, his pulſe was quick, and his ſkin hot. I preſcribed two ſcruples of rheubarb, and thin gruel. 2d, He had an indifferent night; he frequently belched his mouth full of ill taſted ſtuff; he was ſomewhat deaf, and returned indiſtinct anſwers, he craved, his cheeks were fluſhed, and

and his pulſe was rather quicker than natural, and irregular. I gave him ten grains of ipecacoan, and allowed him a little wine.

3d, He complained conſtantly of an ill taſte, and clamminess in his mouth which he was very anxious to get rid of; his tongue in the middle was of a Pomegranate colour, ſurrounded with a black line, and a clean margin or edge he was very giddy; he had frequent looſe ſtools, conſtant tremors, an inordinate craving, a continual thirſt, and was very weak. I ordered him the ſaline mixture made with the ſal. C. C. wherein the ſalt predominated; with the addition of Tinct. Theb. and red port; at the ſame time I allowed him a nouriſhing diet with wine, and gave him a ſlice of a China orange ſprinkled with ſugar, to ſuck frequently. There was Tinct. Theb. gt. vi, in each doſe of his mixture.

4th, His tongue was clean; he complained leſs of heat, and his pulſe was not ſo quick. In other reſpects he was the ſame; and ſeemed to ſleep more than he would allow. I continued his medicines and diet.

5th, His purging without gripes was ſtill troubleſome; and a prickly heat like eruption appeared about his neck and breaſt. I preſcribed Pulv. Rad. Rhei, gr. x. Pulv. Ipecacoan. gr. ii. m. fiat. pulv. matutino ſumendus. The powder puked him gently, and gave him ſeveral ſtools. P. M. his pulſe was more regular, and his skin cool; but his tongue was dry; he ſighed deeply when he ſpoke; and preferred lying on a cheſt to his hammock.

I ordered him Pulv. Contrayerv. C. gr. x. every eight hours, beſides his medicines every four hours as preſcribed on the 3d, with his wine and diet. By accident I learned that he had been ſomewhat delirious on the nights of the 19th, 20th, and 21ſt, of July, but not afterwards.

6th, He was quiet in the night and ſweated profuſely; his tongue was much cleaner; and he complained only of weakneſs. However, the bad taſte of his mouth, his thirſt, purging, tremors, giddineſs, inordinate craving, his deafneſs, and the fluſhing (with a wildneſs now) of his countenance continued. His urine was high coloured. I ſtill repeated all his medicines, continued his wine, and frequently gave him, without his asking for any thing, a little ſago panada, or a toaſt with wine, cinamon, and ſugar added to them.

7th, He was more peeviſh, being now tired of every thing that he was fond of before I ordered all his medicines, wine and diet, to be continued as before.

8th, He was weak and faintiſh; his pulſe was very unequal; his mouth was dry and clammy; his skin was hot, with a diſagreeable moiſture on it; though he complained of nothing except his purging, and that his ſtools were ſmall I preſcribed as before, and an opiate Tinct. Theb. gt. xv. to be given him at night; and likewiſe a large bliſter to be applied between his ſhoulders.

He

9th, He refted well feemingly, but denied that he had any fleep. At noon his pulfe was very fmall; his fkin was cold; and he had a cold clammy fweat over him. He muttered; fpoke inarticulately; and dozed frequently, but would not acknowledge it, nor afked for any thing. I repeated the pulv. contrayerv. c. with theriac. androm. gr. v. every fix hours, and gave him a large fpoonful of the following julap every two hours. ℞. tinct. ferp. virg. ℥iv. fp. vol. arom. ʒifs. aq. fimp. ℥viii. facch. alb. ad gratum faporem. I applied large blifters to the internal parts of his thighs, and continued his wine diet. p. m. he made but one ftool, though his blifters all acted properly, and he feemed rather better—he felt no pain any where.

10th, He refted very well apparently in the night. His pulfe was more regular, his fkin was moift, and moderately warm; his purging was abated, and he complained of his blifters paining him. I omitted the theriac and julap, continued the contrayerva as before, and repeated the following draught every hour. ℞. tinct. cort. peruv. Huxham tinct. rad. ferp. virg. ana ʒi. aq. fimp. ℥i. facch. alb. q. f. fiat hauftus: and likewife his diet as before.

11th, He was eafy but did not fleep in the night; and though he was ftill feverifh and his tongue dry, he complained only of weaknefs, and was hungry. I ordered two ounces of a ftrong decoction of the bark with a little wine and his former diet. p. m. he had only one ftool in the day; was in good fpirits. and in every refpect better. The eruption now increafed about his neck and breaft.

12th, He had a good night, complained much of his blifters in the day, and of great weaknefs. His tongue was moift, and he had very little fever. I repeated his decoction and diet.

13th, He was a little feverifh; a. m. he took his decoction. p. m. He had no fever on him, and complained of his weaknefs and the tremors only.

14th, He was much better, and took his decoction with wine every hour regularly, and diet.

15th, 16th, 17th, 18th, and 19th, He continued to recover. I prefcribed as on the 11th.

20th, He took the decoction every two hours only; on the 21ft day he took it four times, and afterwards morning and evening, until the 26th day of the fever when he returned quite well to his duty.

Six men died on the voyage. The Anomalous cafe; four with the dyfentry, and the man with the mortification.

C H A P. IV.

Remarks on particular Diseases.

Section I.

On the Rhumatiſm.

IN the three voyages we only had twenty nine rheumatic patients, moſt of whoſe caſes were chronical, and yielded to cathartícks, ſmall doſes of calomel and jalap, with a little camphor added thereto, to prevent the mouth from being affected. Sometimes bliſters were applied to the parts, but more frequently they were only rubbed ſeveral times a day with the ol. terebinth. and covered with flannel.

I cured one man who was much troubled with it in one of his wriſts, elbow, and ſhoulder, the ſecond voyage, by rubbing the parts well a few times, with a liquid which Captain Collingwood got from a Gentleman in Jamaica, (who is ſince dead) to rub his limbs with when he was attacked with the gout; which was ſerviceable to him often in allaying the pain. What it was compounded of I know not, but the Gentleman aſſured Captain Collingwood, that it was made from herbs, and had always relieved him when he had been laid up in terrible fits of the gout. It was clear as water, and he deſired it might be always warmed in a baſon, or cup placed in hot water, before it was uſed. In rubbing it on, it leathered ſomewhat, and made the part look red afterwards, and break out in a ſmall eruption. He called it vegetable cream.

The rhumatiſm of laſt Auguſt was acute, of which the patients were more numerous than they were all the firſt voyage. I treated it therefore nearly as acute fevers are managed in a cold climate. A little blood was taken from the patient, a purge adminiſtred and repeated as was neceſſary; and I gave them with ſage tea, or barley water, from thirty to five and forty drops of Huxham's eſſence of antimony, morning and evening; or eight grains of camphor, or two ſpoonfulls of a ſalution of gum guaiac, with ſal. nitre in rum, and a light diet. The ſolution of the gum promoted the alvine diſcharges, as well as a free perſpiration: but unleſs the patient drank plentifully, it was apt to occaſion a ſlight dyſuria. The topical applications were the ſame as in the chronical caſes.

I have known an emetick to be of very great ſervice in a lumbago, when bleeding and purges both repeated, together with ſudorificks had proved ineffectual.

Section II.

On Ulcers.

WITH refpect to ulcers, when they were either of long ftanding, or were very large and foul, as was frequently the cafe, I never found any application whatever really ferviceable in reducing them to a healing condition, until the habit of body was firft mended. That I always effected by repeated purges, with which calomel was joined; abftinence from falt provifions and fpirits; keeping the limb in a horizontal pofture; and giving plenty of the bark in fubftance, fometimes adding elixir of vitriol thereto, and continuing it until the ulcer was healed. Whether the applications to the ulcers were warm digeftives; the precipitate dreffing; dry lint, or cataplafms, &c. by the method I have mentioned, they foon difcharged a laudable pus, diminifhed furprifingly, and put on a healing appearance: after which common dreffings were made ufe of only.

But it is to be obferved, that fcorbutick ulcers are not claffed with thofe which I have been fpeaking of. The proper method of treating them is fet forth at large in Doctor Lind's treatife on the fcurvy.

Section III.

On the Venereal Difeafe.

I Purpofely omitted taking any notice of patients who had the Venereal Difeafe, either in the meteorological journal, or review of the fick lift, becaufe that difeafe is neither endemick, nor epidemick, but is contracted in all countries, and feafons, either by immediate contact with a difeafed perfon, or the matter difcharged from one that is difeafed being inferted into wounds, or fores of well people, or from the matter being applied to, or rubbed upon fome very fine, or delicate part of a found perfon. By one or other of which ways, healthy people in all places, of every age and fex, may be infected, though not with equal readinefs at all times.

Befides it is now become fo univerfal, that the method of curing it, which is generally by mercurials, is almoft well known every where. As coadjutants to mercurials, decoctions of farfaparilla, and the woods are added, particularly in poxes. Bougies, in the cafes of old fufferers, frequently become neceffary in the cure.

Some

Some practitioners, with great confidence, recommend compofitions to prevent infection from libidinous contact; but of thofe compofitions, or their effects, I acknowledge myfelf ignorant.

Seamen now a days indeed, on board of his Majefty's fhips, are fo full of faving their fifteen fhillings, * that from their taking medicines of each others prefcriptions, and their putting off time in that manner, three of every four of them who complained on board of the Rainbow were poxes. But in a good habit of body, after having given a fingle dofe of phyfick—for I do not imagine that it is often neceffary to take away blood—when the patient complained in proper time, and was afterwards temperate in his living, I very feldom failed in curing a recent gonorrhæa with the following pill, adminiftred every night, without the affiftance of any thing elfe than demulcent drink, and abftinence from falt meat. R. Calomel, pp. Rad. Jalap. Pulv. a gr. ii. panis mica madida fiat pilula, omni nocte fumenda.

In hot climates it will often be neceffary to unite Camphor with Mercurials, when they are continued any time; or to adminifter Camphor internally when the ointment is rubbed in, to prevent a falivation from being brought on. I have known a perfon to be thrown into a deep falivation when—to my knowledge—he had only taken five grains of Calomel in two days—two grains and a half one day, and the other two and a half the day following.

Section IV.

A Table *fhewing all the Difeafes, and the number of Patients of each Difeafe in the three different Voyages of the Rainbow.*

The firft column contains the number of patients who died on board; the fecond contains the number of patients of each difeafe; and the third expreffes the different difeafes.

The

---

* That fum they are obliged to pay out of their wages to the Surgeon for curing them of the Venereal Difeafe.

No. of Patients who died.	No of the Patients of each Disease.	The different DISEASES of the three Voyages of his Majeſty's Ship RAINBOW to the Coaſt of *Africa*, in the Years 1772, 1773, and 1774.
	62	Remitting fevers—a number of them mild—eſpecially thoſe which happen'd the two laſt voyages.
	11	Intermitting fevers—including the relapſed remitting fevers.
	1	Slow nervous fever.
	11	Catarrhous fevers.
	169	Slight fevers, including headachs, nauſeæ, colds, and ſuppreſſed perſpirations in hot climates.
	36	Slight fevers, including colds, headachs, and indiſpoſitions in a cold climate.
3	3	Anomalous caſes.
9	96	Dyſentery—many of them were mild and relapſes.
	28	Diarrhœæ.
	17	Bellyachs.
	1	Quinſey.
	4	Sore throats.
	16	Coughs.
	4	Aſthma—one caſe relapſed three times; he came from the Weaſel.
	1	Hectick.
1	1	Vomica.
1	1	Hemoptoſis.
	1	Hemorrhage.
	29	Rheumatiſm, including lumbago, and muſcular pains.
	1	Gout.
	30	Scurvy, including the ſcorbutick ulcers.
	1	Scrophula.
	2	Hypochondria.
	1	Epilepſy.
	1	Deafneſs
	4	Opthalmia.
	1	Dimneſs of ſight.
	2	Suffuſions, which follow opthalmiæ.
	2	Nephritis.
	4	Hæmorrhoides.
	10	Eruptions.
	2	Eryſipelas.
	2	Excoriations.
	3	Scalds.
	4	Strains.
	47	Contuſions.
	5	Wounds.
	3	Fractures.
	10	Inflammations.
	1	Parotis.
	7	Abſceſſes.
	5	Guinea worms—one of them relapſed ſeveral times.]
1	1	Mortification.
	9	Ulcers.
	1	Fiſtula in ano.
	21	Lame—ſlight complaints chiefly.
	1	Weak.
2	2	Accidents.
17	675	Total.—Beſides venereal patients, common ulcers, and ſlight complaints.

PART IV.

A Practical Account of the FEVER and DYSENTERY.

CHAPTER I.

OF THE REMITTING FEVER.

SECTION I.

Arrangement of the Subject.

ALTHOUGH my design does not render it necessary that I should insert a general history of any of the diseases which fell under my observation on board of the Rainbow, yet as the Remitting Fever and the Dysentery were by far the most frequent and dangerous diseases that happened, it may not be altogether improper to give a more particular account of them, and of the method in which I treated them.

It is true, I have already given a very exact account of the Remitting Fever which occurred on board of the Weasel; and indeed I may even venture to say, that it is a valuable one, because, as I have before observed, nature had, in a manner, her own course throughout the Fever, from my not having bark to administer in a proper quantity. But, besides other circumstances which produced a great difference between the Weasel's and the Rainbow's Fever, it will be agreeable to my Readers to observe what a stricking contrast there was between the events of both, which speaks much more powerfully in favour of the bark—as it was liberally made use of in curing the latter—than any oratory whatever possibly could.

I shall therefore, first describe the symptoms of the Fever; secondly, describe two *anomalous* cases; thirdly, offer some observations on the Fever; fourthly, insert the method of cure; and lastly, set down a number of the cases,—dividing those different heads into Sections. With respect to the account of the Dysentery, I have nearly adhered to the same order.

I shall

I ſhall not puzzle myſelf about all the different appellations which are beſtowed on the Remitting Fever, according to the different types of its periods; for I ſuppoſe if a practitioner is only careful to watch his patients, and obſerve attentively the commencement, advancement, height, and declenſion of the paroxyſm, with the particular ſymptoms, ſo as that he may be enabled to preſcribe for them with propriety, I think it will hardly be a matter of much conſequence whether he always juſtly adapts Semitertian according to Hoffman's or Celſus's manner.

However, I would not wiſh to be underſtood that I condemn ſuch accurate and nice diſtinctions. But a practitioner muſt be a long time converſant with the Fever, before he becomes acquainted with the regular operations of nature, from, ſeemingly ſuch various and contrary ways; or be able to comprehend them ſufficiently to apply thoſe diſtinctions with any degree of preciſion. Beſides, there is hardly a Phyſician, who if he was called upon to viſit a patient in the firſt paroxyſm of a Remitting Fever, could tell with certainty whether it would be a ſimple, double, triple or ſemitertian, unleſs he continued with his patient until the period was ended; and even then he could ſcarcely aſcertain what appearance the Fever would put on in its next period, becauſe various circumſtances might concur to alter the types thereof, from what they were in the firſt period—even ſuppoſing no medicine had been given in either. So great then muſt be the difficulty of attaining a perfect knowledge of applying ſuch diſtinctions, not to mention thoſe which are farther made from the ſymptoms.

In the ſubſequent account, I ſhall therefore ſtill retain the term of a Remitting Fever, whatever types the periods may put on, becauſe that is perfectly underſtood by every practitioner without any further explanation. Beſides, it is already done by many learned and able Phyſicians; eſpecially by Sir *John Pringle*, in his Obſervations on the Diſeaſes of the Army; Doctor *Lind* in his book on Hot Climates; and Mr *Cleghorn*, in his Treatiſe on the Diſeaſes of Minorca, who is remarkably particular on that head.

However, inſtead of obſerving the diurnal occurrences in the following account, I ſhall be more particular with regard to the periods; the paroxyſms; and the ſymptoms happening in each of them; becauſe, though in fact it will amount to one and the ſame thing, I think I will be more clearly underſtood by ſo doing, which is all I wiſh for.

SEC.

SECTION II.

The Remitting Fever described.

THE Remitting Fever generally began with a chillineſs; a ſevere headach; a ſickneſs at ſtomach; and pains in all the bones, but eſpecially in the loins.

But ſome drooped ſeveral days before they were bad, were chilly, and hot alternately, and had rigours, the cold fit continuing twelve hours; ſome without any ſenſation of chillineſs, were at once ſeized with burning heat, profuſe ſweats, and violent headachs. Together with the general ſymptoms, ſome were ſeized with a fixed pain in the ſide, or breaſt, affecting the reſpiration; pains in the ſhoulders; pains over the eyes; pain and oppreſſion about the præcordia with wandering pains, and univerſal ſoreneſs, and uneaſineſs. Some were ſeized with a nauſea, a bad taſte in the mouth, with a vomiting of bilious matter, ſevere vomitings and purgings, a hemorrhage at the noſe, watery eyes, a headach, and univerſal illneſs, with great anxiety and deſpondency, a ſudden giddineſs and faintneſs only, and an obſtinate coſtiveneſs; the ſkins of ſome, but particularly the palms of their hands, were exceſſively hot and dry; and their thirſt vehement.

Their pulſes varied according to the manner in which they were ſeized; in ſome caſes they were ſlow and weak, in ſome they were ſmall and quick, and in others they were quick and ſtrong.

In all theſe various ways did the fever commence. But if they were at firſt ſeized with a chillineſs or rigours, a burning heat, great uneaſineſs and breathleſſneſs ſucceeded; the headach and pain of the loins became much more violent; ſome of their countenances were greatly fluſhed; their eyes much inflamed; the reaching was more troubleſome, and their thirſt intenſe. Thus they continued, until a profuſe ſweat broke out, generally, which relieved them of their complaints, more or leſs: for in whatever manner they were firſt ſeized, except in the anomalous caſes to be deſcribed, the paroxyſm terminated in a greater or leſs degree of ſweat; and that varied much both as to its duration and violence amongſt them.

In the remiſſion, they all complained of great laſſitude and weakneſs, of pains, and ſoreneſs of their bones, giddineſs, and loſs of appetite. Their pulſes were rather more languid than a healthy perſon's; and though their ſkins were now much cooler, they continued very thirſty; but either as to its calmneſs or duration, it varied amongſt them, as much as the preceding paroxyſm had done. Indeed, to ſuch a degree did they both vary, that not in any two patients were they exactly ſimilar.

Some after having ſweated a little only, which hardly alleviated their complaints, continued quite uneaſy, until the next paroxyſm, by terminating in a profuſe ſweat, relieved them; ſo that they in a manner had two paroxyſms before there was a remiſſion.

The ſecond paroxyſm, which in ſome patients was preceded by rigours, was in every one more violent than the firſt. The headach and lumbago were particularly vehement; the latter in ſome, extending quite round the abdomen, which was painful when touched, and very tenſe; ſome were delirious; pains of the breaſt and ſide were very acute, the latter extending as low as the leg; ſome had great oppreſſion about the præcordia, bilious vomitings and purgings, and idle notions, with fear of falling aſleep, were very troubleſome, as was a hæmorrhage at the noſe, and a ſenſation of chillineſs during the whole paroxyſm. Their pulſes were irregular, and their ſkins impreſſed a diſagreeable ſenſation on the fingers. In a few caſes I obſerved, as before, inſtead of one, there were two paroxyſms, or a double one. But every one in whoſe caſe a remiſſion was evident, had two paroxyſms within the firſt period, or forty-eight hours, a few only exceeding that time by three or four hours. In two patients there was only one paroxyſm which continued nearly the whole period. As to the paroxyſms, the firſt was of longeſt duration in ſome, and the ſecond in others; but neither of them exceeded twenty-four hours, except the two mentioned.

The preceding paroxiſm left them all very weak, anxious, and dejected, with a burning heat in the palms of their hands, and ſoles of their feet; a loſs of taſte, or a bitter taſte in their mouths, and inſatiable thirſt. The remiſſion continued longer, and was more diſtinct in ſome than in other caſes. With one perſon it was nearly the whole period, which proved to be only a very deceitful receſſion, for he had two very violent paroxyſms the period following.

In the ſecond period, a few patients had one long and two ſhort paroxyſms---ſome one long and one ſhort---and others had but one paroxyſm, which was of longer duration in ſome caſes than in others. So much they continued to vary, and even in the ſame patient the hour of commencement was altered; and in the paroxyſms, which were ſtill preceded by chillineſs, beſides the former ſymptoms, there were troubleſome coughs; during which eſpecially the head ſeemed to open and ſhut; a ſtricture and pain over the eyes and at the bottoms of the orbits; great difficulty in breathing from weight and oppreſſion about the præcordia, together with faintneſs; frequent and deep ſighs; the abdomen was ſwelled and conſtipated: ſome had a diſuria, and the urine was very ſmall in quantity and quite turbid, which indeed occurred in the former period in one caſe; a bilious vomiting and purging in the place of a paroxyſm; and a very profuſe hæmorrhage at the nose; their dread of falling asleep; and the anxiety and despondency were greater; the delirium was more general; some of their tongues were brown and rough; and their countenances sallow and fallen.

The paroxysms in a few cases ended with bilious stools and a moderate sweat; but generally, as before, in a profuse sweat. One or two had a very mild period. During the remissions, which as usual varied in their duration; they were all much weaker; nothing pleased their taste; none of them would swallow any food; their giddiness was greater; and some of them were faint-ish on the least motion.

In the third, as well as in the former periods, some patients had only one, some two, some had three, and some even four paroxysms, which were preceded by a griping. Many new and more dangerous symptoms appeared too. They who were not seemingly so bad hitherto, were much weaker, and their spirits more depressed than others whose paroxysms had been apparently more violent; a coma; an immoderate discharge of urine: some who had no pains before, were seized with acute ones, and straitness in the sides and breast, much pain about the scrobiculum cordis, with great anxiety, depression, and despondency. Their pains who had any before, now extended more and more. Coughs were more general, with a wheezing and great difficulty of breathing. Partial, angry, prickly heat, like eruptions, appeared. The tongues in some were white and dry; in others husky, and the teeth covered with black sordes; a pain about the throat, which rendered deglutition difficult; the flushing of their countenances was greater; their pulses were more irregular, and all the other symptoms were greatly increased. There was an obvious privation of the senses, and of all motion, except a convulsive one about the mouth, cold extremities, clammy cold sweats, a tremulous thready pulse, and a subsultus tendinum; the impression on the fingers from feeling the pulse was more disagreeable, and continued longer.

The remissions in the third period were very imperfect; and, besides the former complaints, which were all severer, they were extremely weak and quite faint; but the remission preceding the fourth period was much more distinct, and of longer duration that any one before.

In the fourth period, a few only had two paroxysms, which were mild; and several had none at all; but they still had a constant small fever, with giddiness; a lumbago; prostration of strength, and faintness; and a few had cold sweats on them. Their medicines puked some, and purged a greater number. Eruptions broke out about their mouths.

Even in the fifth period, one or two patients had very slight paroxysms.

The preceding is a very exact account of all the bad Remitting Fevers which occurred during the three voyages, except two cases which I shall describe under the term of *Anomalous*, before I proceed to make any observati-

ons,

ons, as they differed widely from all the reſt, notwithſtanding they were one and the ſame Fever.

Sec. III.

Anomalous Cases *of the* Remitting Fever, *in which the Symptoms are inſerted diurnally, for obvious Reaſons.*

MR. aged about forty years, a ſtrong man of a middle ſize, and florid complexion, who very ſeldom in his life had been ailing, complained, after drooping a few days, on the evening of the 28th of April, lat. at noon 0.1°. 12″ S. of a headach; pains in all his limbs and bones, * with thirſt. 29th and 1ſt of his illneſs, a. m. he was ſick at his ſtomach; his former complaints were rather more troubleſome; his ſkin was diſagreeable to the touch, though not extremely hot; his pulſe was quicker than in a natural ſtate; his tongue white; with a proſtration of his ſtrength and ſpirits. P. M. his puke operated. He was very anxious and much afraid.

2d. He had a bad night's reſt; he was coſtive; his head was light, and rather giddy; he wandered a little; he was nice about trifles; his urine was high coloured with whitiſh fibres in it; his pulſe was irregular; but he had no ſevere complaint, though he was greatly afraid of dying.

3d. His countenance was fluſhed and rather wild after having been much troubled with inquietude in the night, and fear of falling aſleep from idle notions plaguing him; his head was more light and giddy, notwithſtanding he had a number of copious fetid ſtools, and complained little. His pulſe and ſkin continued much the ſame; and his urine was paler without cloud or ſediment.

4th. He paſſed a very reſtleſs night; his ſkin was quite dry; ſometimes he had a pain for a little in his right leg; he complained very little, only by expreſſing his deſpondency; and his urine was ſtill more pale P. m. there was a ſmall cloud at the top of the glaſs, but in the night there was no ſign of one in his urine, which was very pale. He had two copious ſtools; and from his looks, ſpectators imagined there was very little the matter with him.

5th. He had an exceeding uneaſy night; he ſighed frequently; his pulſe was ſofter and ſlower than natural; his ſkin was dry and rather hot; his tongue was white and ſcabrous; and his urine was pale with filaments in it. When he was quiet, he lay with his hands folded over the thorax, and frequently clapped the ſcrobiculum cordis with his right hand; and when he was ſpoke to he raiſed himſelf ſuddenly upon one of his elbows. P. m. He com-

* This was his own Phraſe.

complained very little, ſlept for a ſhort time, and awoke frightened; he had a copious ſtool, and his urine was full of clear, ſmall air bubbles.

6. He was more reſtleſs than he had been any night; he wandered much, talked conſtanly of dying; his ſkin was dry, hot, and diſagreeable to the touch; a prickly heat like eruption broke out on his breaſt and neck, and his urine was of a bright amber colour without either cloud or ſediment. P. m. He wandered more, and was extremely reſtleſs. At midnight he was quiet, and had no complaint, but he ſwallowed his medicine in an unuſual manner, refuſed to take all of it, and his ſpirits were ſeemingly very much agitated: after which he lay down as to ſleep, but died at 5 a. m. on the 7th day of his illneſs. ——He had a copious ſtool the 6th day.----From firſt to laſt there was no remiſſion. For the manner in which he was treated, ſee the review of the ſick liſt May 1772.

M. F. aged about ſixteen, never had been in a hot climate before, after drooping a conſiderable time, complained the 31ſt July p. m. lat. at noon 34° 58″ of a loſs of appitite, headach, and ſickneſs at ſtomach. His pulſe too was quicker than natural. 2d Day of his illneſs, his complaints were rather eaſier, but he was ſtill feveriſh. 3. He would not take the medicines which were preſcribed for him; ſaid that he was pretty well, and would go on deck. 4. He made no complaints, nor would take his medicine, though he was entreated. 5. He complained of being unwell, and very coſtive. P m. He was well purged. 6. He found himſelf better, though he was ſtill a little feveriſh, and had no moiſture on his ſkin; but he was not thirſty.

7. He got cold, complained again of his headach, and ſickneſs at ſtomach. His tongue was white, his ſkin hot and dry, and his pulſe was quick and hard. P. m. His pulſe was much quicker and harder, nevertheleſs he became faintiſh upon loſing about five ounces of blood. 8. He raved in the night, his pulſe was ſofter and not ſo quick; his headach, and ſickneſs at ſtomach continued; his ſkin was hot and dry, and he was now thirſty.

9. He was very irregular in his living. A. m. he complained of his bliſter only which prevented him from ſleeping in the night; he was very giddy when out of bed, p. m, and began to rave. His medicine procured him a number of copious ſtools.

10. He ſlept, and perſpired a little, but was not refreſhed. His ſkin became hot and dry; he complained of nothing, nor had either thirſt or appetite; his tongue was white, and a diſagreeable ſenſation remained on the fingers for ſome time after feeling his pulſe. P. m. He was very reſtleſs, delirious, he looked frequently at his hands, and bit his nails. 11 He was quieter and ſlept two hours a. m; he awoke and vomited what he had eat the preceding day at noon, as entire and indigeſted as when he ſwallowed it; again dropped to ſleep, but denied that he had ſlept any when he awoke; he was more

more delirious, and restless, particularly with his hands; his legs and feet were cold, yet he complained of nothing. P. m. After taking Doctor James's powder, he had a profuse clammy sweat on him, made some high coloured urine, which deposited a lateritious sediment, and had several convulsive rigours, which continued some minutes.

12. He had a very bad night, being troubled with great inquietude; he had a profuse clammy sweat on him again from Doctor James's powder, but was no way relieved. P. m. He roared out, though he denied that he had any pain, and had convulsive twitches at times. At night his skin was dry and hot, his pulse was soft and irregular, and his tongue was swelled, white, and foul.

13. He had no rest in the night, though he perspired; his pulse was very small; he was very weak, but sensible, and eat a little several times; his tongue was covered with a black coat, he spat a little blood, and had an involuntary discharge of urine--whether the last symptom proceeded from his blisters or not, is a doubt with me.

14. He spent the night as usual. A. m he spat a little more blood, and a few drops fell from his nose; the involuntary discharge of urine continued; he had partial sweats; his skin was very disagreeable to the touch, and his pulse was very small and irregular. The abdomen though constipated was neither swelled, tense, nor painful upon being pressed; yet he seemed to feel great pain upon introducing the pipe of the clyster syringe into the anus with the greatest care; and a very small quantity of the injection could be thrown up at a time, from an obstruction in the rectum. At 8 p. m. he died of a return of his convulsive rigours.

SECTION IV

Observations on the Remitting Fever.

THE odd days 3, 5, 7, and so on, were remarkable for more paroxysms happening on them, for their continuing longer, and for their violence.

The cessation of the fever and symptoms on the 3d and 4th days was very deceitful; for an exacerbation of both returned on the 5th. The calm which happened on the 6th day, and was followed by an exacerbation of both fever and symptoms on the 7th, proved fatal. Imminent danger attended an obstinate costiveness throughout the fever. Despondency was an exceeding dangerous symptom. The case proved extremely bad wherein the patient was seized with sudden giddiness and faintness. The sickness at stomach which continued until the 11th day was mortal. Spitting a little blood, and a few drops falling from the nose, proved mortal, as *Cleghorn* justly observed. Nor was the event more favourable where there was no natural evacuation, but such as was forced by medicines Urine which was high coloured, in ſmall quantity, and depoſited a lateritious ſediment, proved fatal. The caſe was equally dangerous when the urine was pale, depoſited no ſediment, but contained filaments or ſmall clear air bubbles.

But of all the prognoſticks, which I have yet been able to form in remitting fevers, that was the moſt fatal---when the patient thought himſelf too well to be in bed, but was not clever, as he expreſſed himſelf; and when he was anxious, uneaſy, and had hardly any complaint, though he was evidently not recovering. Roaring out without having any pain, and convulſive rigours, followed the uſe of Doctor James's fever powder, on the 11th day in the laſt anomalous caſe; but I will not take upon me to ſay that theſe ſymptoms were the conſequence of that *myſterious* powder; notwithſtanding I muſt ſay in juſtice to the publick, that upon the faireſt trials, which I have repeatedly made between that powder and the Tartar Emetick, given in ſimple water only, the latter always proved to be the moſt effectual remedy, though it is on a moderate calculation a thouſand times cheaper than the former.

With reſpect to the critical days, one died on the 7th, and the other on 14th. All the other caſes were cured by bark.

SECTION V.

Method of Cure.

LETTING more or leſs blood in the beginning of remitting fevers, is not only practiſed, but recommended as abſolutely neceſſary by many eminent phyſicians; whilſt others of equal eminence, from their inculcating the utmoſt degree of caution, and recommending the ſtricteſt frugality in taking away blood, ſeem tacitly to condemn the practice altogether.

When the firſt or ſecond Paroxſyms are extremely violent, the pulſe ſtrong and quick, or ſtrong and much oppreſſed, the eyes much inflamed, the ſkin extremely hot, when there are fixed acute pains about the thorax; the patient too very athletic, and lately arrived from a cold climate---eſpecially, when moſt of theſe circumſtances concur in one caſe---it muſt certainly be neceſſary to take away blood. However, ſuch a caſe will hardly ever be met with upon the coaſt of Africa, becauſe the people are ſome time in a warm climate before they can reach it, conſequently the pores of the ſkin being ſufficiently opened, the tenſion or rigidity of the fibres, how great ſoever it might be before, is neceſſarily removed, which obviates ſuch ſymptoms, if they are taken bad. And notwithſtanding, when there is an apparent urgency for the operation, it will rarely be found to anſwer any good purpoſe. Indeed this will afford matter of no great wonder, if it be conſidered that the *vis vitæ* is ſunk, or oppreſſed in a much greater pro-

portion

portion than their *folids* are relaxed, who are feized with fevers foon after their arrival in hot climates, particularly on the coaft of Africa, where the air, efpecially in the fickly parts, is always hazy and moift, notwithftanding the fun fhines, with heavy dews in the night, which amazingly depreffes the fpirits even of thofe who are well, as I have taken notice of in the meteorological journal,

Before I went on that coaft, I learned from obfervation in the Weft Indies, and at Penfacola, that the taking away of blood in remitting fevers, was hardly of any fervice; and that, I own, had greater weight with me than any theory whatever. I muft own too I am of opinion, that the benefit which fome practitioners attribute to opening the venæ faphenæ has been chiefly owing to the pediluvium made ufe of upon the occafion and not to the quantity of blood which was taken away.

For thofe reafons, I was very cautious in ufing my lancet in the cure of the fever; and although I never did let blood * but in the St. Jago fever, when we were only juft arrived in a hot climate, in two cafes of the Sierra Leon fever, and in the laft anomalous cafe---for which I thought I had fufficient ground, as we were then in latitude, 40° 03″---yet none of them were the better for it, nor could bear the lofs of a very few ounces without becoming faintifh, except one of the cafes of the Sierra Leon fever, and he was fubject to maniacal complaints. I ordered twelve ounces only to be taken from him; and upon weighing it afterwards, there were full fixteen ounces taken away; however, he bore it well, and to a great advantage.

From hence, the great impropriety of paying much attention to the moft fpecious theory in favour of blood letting in remitting fevers of hot climates, is fufficiently obvious.

Any precaution that might have appeared neceffary for me to have taken with my patients during the different ftages of the firft paroxyfm---efpecially the cold one when it happened, was prevented by their feldom complaining until it was quite over.

The firft ftep therefore, which I generally took towards the cure, was to give an emetick. But though nature points out the neceffity for that evacuation, either by reachings to vomit, or a ficknefs at ftomach, fome practitioners wholly condemn it. However, their objections, as they are only the offspring of a favourite theory, do not deferve ferious attention. The quantity of bile which is always brought up therewith, not to mention the other advantages which it is productive of, will always render it neceffary in the opinion of them who are guided by cool reflection.

If

* The remitting fever of December 1772, is no exception to this rule, becaufe it happened in a cold climate.

If I did not ſee my patient during the firſt paroxyſm, I always gave it before the ſecond commenced; otherwiſe I ordered it either in the cold or hot ſtage, but omitted giving it until the paroxyſm was ended, if the ſweat had broke out before I was called; preſcribing in ſuch caſes, only plenty of ſub-acid diluting drink, neither hot, nor quite cold, to promote it, and the urinary diſcharge, as well as to allay the patient's thirſt. When there were no ſuch regular ſtages during the paroxyſm, as too generally was the caſe, I gave the vomit as ſoon as I was called upon, after the ſame manner as in the Weaſels fever, (See page 16th) which was wrought off with warm water, barley water, or very thin gruel. Beſides operating by vomit, it likewiſe procured the patient a copious ſtool or two, promoted a free perſpiration, and more ſpeedily terminated the paroxyſm (when it was given in either of the two firſt ſtages thereof) than happened in ſuch caſes as did not complain until the ſweat had broken out; then I only allowed them drink until the remiſſion, when the vomit was adminiſtered.

If it was in the evening they took it, I preſcribed in an hour and an half, or two hours after, a ſaline draught with more or leſs of the eſſen. antimon. according to the age of the patient and other circumſtances, and plenty of ſage tea or barley water, either acidulated, or with ſal. nitr. and his purge the morning following.

But when the vomit was adminiſtered in the morning, whether it procured one or two ſtools, I generally ordered the purge to be given in two hours after its operation; which was an ounce of the ſal. cathart. amar. diſſolved in half a pint of thin gruel or barley water, divided into four parts, and one of them given every half hour; for as the ſtomach was not only loaded with bile, but the inteſtines likewiſe with bilious *Saburra*, I thought that they never could be too ſoon emptied of their noxious contents, which that method always effected in a mild and gentle way; and indeed I found it neceſſary ſometimes to repeat both thoſe evacuations, particularly the purge in the courſe of the fever.

Of all the authors who have publiſhed their ſentiments concerning the method of treating the remmitting fever, which I have met with, though they differ in opinion with reſpect to bleeding and vomiting, not one of them condemns purging; the advantages ariſing therefrom being too obvious to admit of any theoretical diſpute, or a heſitation concerning the propriety of it. Indeed it is aſtoniſhing to ſee the prodigious quantity of fetid and even putrid *colluvies*, which is diſcharged by purges, and ſometimes without their aſſiſtance, to the great relief of the patients. In ſome caſes they never have a ſtool, unleſs laxatives are daily adminiſtered; and what would be the conſequence, if the putrid Saburra was pent up in the inteſtines throughout the fever.

Though

Though purging is abſolutely neceſſary, I apprehend that the moſt dangerous conſequences would enſue from the uſe of *draſtick* purges, I therefore made uſe of no other, than either the ſal. cath. amar. or glauber. generally alone, becauſe manna is by much too expenſive for common uſe on board of his Majeſty's ſhips. Tamarind beverage generally proved not only an agreeable drink, but likewiſe a laxative; by which therefore, too very material advantages were frequently obtained. It no doubt would be moſt proper to adminiſter the purge in a remiſſion, but they were ſo ſhort and imperfect generally, as well as uncertain, that I very ſeldom waited for one; and therefore gave it ſoon after the operation of the emetick was over, as I have already mentioned, or the morning following; and a ſaline draught* with eſſen. antimon. at night.

Notwithſtanding the indifference with which ſaline draughts are made mention of by ſome authors, I found them a moſt uſeful vehicle for the eſſ antimon. or tart. emet.---without one or other of theſe antimonials, I never gave them in the fever---as well as ſerviceable in aſſiſting to allay the thirſt. They were made after the uſual manner, and well diluted, and the antimonials added in ſuch proportions, with or without ſal. nitr. as I judged proper; but in ſome caſes, I preferred the ſp. Mindereri to the draughts to which the antimonials were always joined. I gave a large ſpoonful of one or other of them every hour, or every two hours; and I am certain, that that medicine frequently ſhortened the paroxyſm, by promoting freely the urinary diſcharges, as well as cutaneous. During the remiſſion it was given much ſeldomer. Sometimes I gave camphor, though it ſeldom agreed with the patient in any form, and at others, the pulv. contrayerv. com. but I found them of no material ſervice. When the headach was violent, the tinct. theb. given after Doctor Lind's method, was ſerviceable for a time, eſpecially if the pediluvium was joined to its aſſiſtance; tho for that purpoſe, bliſters were by far the moſt effectual remedy.

However, without bark there was no cure; for the only two who died took none, for the reaſons which I have already mentioned. I always adminiſtered it in ſubſtance, to the quantity of one drachm, one and an half, or two drachms, which I never exceeded for a doſe, nor ever ordered it ſeldomer or oftner than once an hour. Sometimes I gave the tincture along with it; but the doſe was not diminiſhed. When I firſt began giving it, the ſtomach was ſo weak, as not to be able to retain it in water alone, I therefore added either tinct. cort. peruv Huxham, ʒii. a ſpoonful or two of wine, or tinct. theb. gr. x. to every one or two doſes, until the ſtomach thereby acquired ſufficient ſtrength to retain it in water only, which commonly was after ſix or ſeven doſes.

P p Though

* It was always made with vegetable acid when I had it, and likewiſe added to their drink.

Though my manner of giving it, was far from being an elegant one, I have the ſatisfaction to ſay, that it never failed me once, amongſt all the caſes of the remitting fever, wherein I made trial of it on board the Rainbow. I mixed an ounce of the powder in twelve ounces or three gills of ſimple water, and ordered that quantity to be given in eight hours; an ounce and an half was mixed in a pint of water, which was ordered to be taken in the ſame time, when I wanted to give a drachm and a half every hour; and when I ordered two drachms of it every hour, two ounces were mixed up in five gills of water, and given in eight doſes—ſometimes a little elixir of vitriol was added—and the patient's mouth was waſhed with a little of his drink, which he ſwallowed after every doſe. Whatever be the vehicle that it is to be given in on board of a ſhip, it is abſolutely neceſſary to mix it up before it be delivered into the charge of the attendants; for to give it out to them in papers, in ſingle doſes, would not only almoſt employ one perſon conſtantly to weigh them, and make them up, if there were many patients, but the attendants, ſuppoſing they were very careful, would be liable to loſe ſome of the papers wholly, and a part of every one in mixing them up, from the motion of the ſhip; both of which inconveniencies are obviated, by mixing up a quantity at once, and putting it into a bottle, that can be ſafely diſpoſed of ſeveral ways; and let me repeat, that ſuch a precaution, ſimple as it is, is well worth attending to for various reaſons.

As to the time of my beginning to adminiſter it, I thought proper to vary it in different patients; but I never began before the end of the firſt period, or third day. After I did begin, I continued to give it regularly every hour, unleſs the violence of the paroxyſms obliged me to omit a few hours, until I was ſure that there was no danger of the fever returning, and in the night as well as the day For I judged it more expedient to employ the time in adminiſtering the ſure means of ſoon procuring them a quiet and refreſhing ſleep, than to allow them to waſte it in reſtleſs ſlumbers. On board of the Weaſel, in two caſes of the fever, a remiſſion was introduced by ſound ſleep, which never happened in the fever on board of the Rainbow.

The number of doſes was then gradually leſſened to once every two, three, four and ſix hours. After they arrived at a convaleſcent ſtate, I gave them either a ſtrong decoction of the bark, with elix. vitr. or an infuſion thereof with rad. ſerp. virg. gentian. & cort. aurant. in wine, twice or thrice a day until they were perfectly recovered, which was in an amazing ſhort time, conſidering how every ill many of them were.

During the cure, I ſometimes added the ſal. cath. amar. with the bark, when the patient was coſtive, though it very ſeldom failed to procure one or more copious ſtools at firſt; and when it brought on a diarrhæa, I added the

the tinct. theb. along with it, which was very ſeldom the caſe; or if vomiting happened therefrom.*

The dietary part had no ſhare in the cure, except in ſome very mild caſes, for I never could get the ſick to take any thing of food, unleſs their drink and medicine be reckoned ſuch, until the fever was ſubdued. I am therefore ſurprized at ſome practitioners of eminence, who ſpeak of breakfaſt, dinner, and ſupper, for their patients during the fever, as if they could really be perſuaded or prevailed upon to take regular meals. After they began to take a little food, till they were pretty well recovered, inſtead of getting them---or the ſick in any acute diſeaſe---to take their meals regularly, I was contented always to indulge them every now and then with a little, as they had an inclination.

The diet for the ſick on board of his Majeſty's ſhips, as well as for the well people, as Doctor Lind has obſerved, far excels what is allowed in any other ſervice. The former is entirely under the direction of the ſurgeon, and conſiſts chiefly of ſago, rice gruel, water gruel, and panado, to which wine and ſpices are occaſionally added, † and portable broth with barley, beſides what the captain and officers ſend them from their tables; and fiſh, when they can be caught with ſcenes, or hooks and lines---every ſhip being ſupplied with one or two of the former, and a proportion of the latter, according to the number of her men, and the ſtation ſhe is ſent upon.

Before I cloſe this head, I cannot help making mention of a circumſtance which I obſerved amongſt the ſick people, when the fever raged on board; and though it may ſeem trivial to ſome folks, it is ſeldom to be met with amongſt ſeamen, or perhaps ſhore patients——A viſible ſatisfaction appeared in their countenances, when I began to give them the bark; and even they, with whom it diſagreed, took it with chearfulneſs—This was certainly owing to their own obſervation of its ſalutary effects, in the caſes of their fellow ſufferers.

SECTION VI

Caſes of the Fever.

CASE I *At St. Jago.*

JOHN Everet, marine, aged about thirty, on February the 3d, 1772, when ſentinel over the water on the booms, the night after anchoring in Praya Bay,

* For further obſervations concerning the bark, ſee the poſtſcript.

† Flower and water well boiled, thin, with a little wine, ſugar and cinnamon added to it, makes a good meſs.

Bay, at the iſland of St. Jago, was ſeized with a chillineſs, which was ſucceeded by alternate heats and rigours, that continued eight hours; he became very hot then; he had a vehement headach; his bones, particularly his loins, pained him much; and he was very thirſty. A profuſe ſweat broke out on him, in about three hours after, which eaſed him, he ſaid. At noon following,

1ſt Of his illneſs, a paroxyſm returned without any chillineſs, and p. m. he complained of a violent headach; all his other complaints were much ſeverer; and his pulſe was full and quick. Near ten ounces of blood were took from him, which made him faintiſh, and an emetick preſcribed for him in four hours after, that brought much bile off his ſtomach, gave him ſeveral copious ſtools, and promoted a free perſpiration; nevertheleſs, the paroxyſm was not ended before midnight.

2d. He was pretty cool, but complained of great proſtration of ſtrength; univerſal pain; and loſs of appetite. I preſcribed the elix. vitr. twice, and a ſaline draught with eſſen. antimon. and ſubacid drink at night.

3d. At midnight a proxyſm returned, and remitted at 6 a. m. Another paroxyſm returned at noon which continued only about four hours; and though neither of them were ſo violent as the preceding ones, he complained of much greater weakneſs, and giddineſs in the remiſſions; and his pulſe was ſmall and quick. I repeated his draught as the preceding night, every four hours.

4th. A. m. he had a ſhort paroxyſm preceded by rigours; he was very feveriſh, thirſty, and, with his former complaints, had a pain in his right ſide all day. He continued his ſaline medicine as before.

5th. He awoke at four, a. m. in a profuſe ſweat, quite languid, and dejected. I ordered him a drahm of bark every hour. At ten, a. m. his fever and complaints returned with more violence than ever; and the pain of his ſide extended down to his knee. During the paroxyſm he took his antimonial medicine as uſual.

6th. The fever continued all day with burning heat in the palms of his hands and ſoles of his feet. I ordered him tart. emet. gr. $\frac{1}{4}$, every two hours, which purged him ſeveral times.

7th. At midnight a ſhort exacerbation came on, and the fever continued all day. I preſcribed his bark again, with a little elix. vitr. and he took an ounce and a half, which ſat eaſy on his ſtomach.

8th. He complained of weakneſs only, and took the ſame quantity of bark as on the 7th.

9th, 10th, 11th, 12th, 13th, 14th, and 15th. He continued recovering, and took half an ounce of bark daily. On the 16th day he returned well to duty; and took the decoction of bark twice a day for ſome time after.

CASE

CASE II.

Andrew Thompſon, a ſtrong healthy ſeaman, aged about 36 years, was took ill the 3d of February, p. m. while at work on the ſhrouds, but complained only on the 5th, when his headach, and pain of his loins were violent; he was very giddy at times, and his pulſe was quick and full. He had been very hot, and ſweated profuſely from his firſt being ſeized, in Praya Bay, St. Jago. I ordered ten ounces of blood to be taken from him, by which the pulſe was much lowered, and he was faintiſh; an emetick in three hours after; and a ſaline draught with the antimonial at night.

2d Day of his complaining, he reſted very indifferently, and his headach and thirſt ſtill continued; though his loins were eaſier. I preſcribed a doſe of ſalts for him, which operated well. At 4 p. m. an exacerbation came on, and at night he took his antimonial draught with refrigerating drink.

3d. The paroxyſm remitted at midnight. Though his ſkin was pretty cool his headach continued without any inclination for food; and he was very weak and thirſty. The antimonial mixture was ordered him every four hours.

4th. He reſted better, and was eaſy in the morning. At 6 p. m. his fever and complaints returned. I repeated his medicine and drink.

5th. He complained leſs, but his fever and thirſt continued. I ordered him a drachm of the bark every hour, which agreed very well with him.

6th. Weakneſs was his only complaint; and he continued his bark.

7th, and 8th. He took only half an ounce of his bark each day, and would return to his duty the 9th. I ordered him the decoction with elixir of vitriol twice a day, for ſome time after.

CASE III.

The Sierra Leon Fever.

John Stringer, marine, aged about 32, a very lifeleſs creature, who never was in a hot climate before, and had been drooping ſome days, complained on the 27th of February---Lat. at noon, 08° 13″---of a headach, ſickneſs at ſtomach, and univerſal pains. I ordered him an emetick which operated well, and an antimonial draught with acidulated drink at night.

2d. He reſted indifferently, with a weakneſs and ſevere pain in his knees; his thirſt was urgent, his tongue white, and his pulſe fuller and quicker than natural. I preſcribed a doſe of ſalts for him, and the antimonial medicine at night with his drink.

3d. He was much better, but could not tell me either when, or in what manner the fever remitted. However, he complained of weaknefs, of heat in the palms of his hands, and foles of his feet, and of a bad tafte in his mouth. I ordered him the antimonial medicine three times.

4th. He continued better, though he was both feverifh and coftive. I gave him fix drahms of the fal. cath. amar. which purged him; and his draught at night as ufual.

5th, A. m. a fevere paroxyfm returned, he knew not when; his headach was fo violent that it feemed to open and fhut; the pain of his loins was very acute with great proftration of ftrength and fpirits; his tongue was white and foul; and his thirft infatiable. P. m. the fever remitted by a profufe perfpiration, and left him quite languid and giddy, with his ufual complaints feverer. I ordered him a faline draught with tart. emet. gr. fs. every three hours during the paroxyfm, and then his ufual medicine with drink.

6th. He had a very reftlefs night; he generally lay on his back, with his hands folded over the fcrobiculum cordis; where he complained of great oppreffion, and of being extremely weak. He could not tell me when he became worfe. At 6 a. m. there was a fmall remiffion, his tongue was brown and rough, and his countenance fallow and much fallen P. m. he was rather better, and his tongue cleaner. I ordered him his antimonial mixture every four hours, and drink as ufual.

7th. At 4 a. m. a paroxyfm returned with increafed violence, and continued all day; p. m. he raved at times, and had a ftupor on him. A large blifter was applied between his fhoulders, and his medicine repeated as before.

8th. The fever remitted a little in the night, and left him quite languid. I ordered the bark for him, a drachm every hour, which was not regularly adminiftered. 9th. He had a fhort paroxyfm in the night; and continued taking his bark, with elix. vitr. every two hours only, which agreed very well with him, ʒifs. for a dofe. He never had another paroxyfm, though he continued weak until the 20th of April, during which time, he took a great deal of bark.

C A S E IV.

John Wakefield, marine, aged about 40, was feized the fame day as the preceding cafe, at 4 a. m. with a headach, ficknefs at ftomach, and univerfal pains and forenefs. When he complained on the 29th of February, p. m. he found himfelf worfe; both his fpirits and ftrength were much proftrated, his countenance was dejected, and his pulfe was quick and fmall. I prefcribed ſcribed an emetick for him, and an antimonial draught with ſubacid drink at night.

2d Day of his complaining, he had a very indifferent night, all his complaints continued; he had a bitter taſte in his mouth, and was very thirſty. I gave him a doſe of ſalts, which purged him, and his draught at night as before.

3d. At 2 a. m. a violent exacerbation came on; fear and wild notions prevented him from ſleep; he h d a ſtricture and pain over his eyes, and at the bottoms of the orbits; his thirſt was inſatiable, and he raved much. I applied a large bliſter between his ſhoulders, put his feet and legs in warm water, and gave him tart. emet. gr. ſs. in a ſaline draught, with tinct. theb gt. xv. every four hours, and acidulated his drink with lime juice.

4th. About 2 a. m. there was a ſlight remiſſion; yet his thirſt continued, his tongue was white and rough, the palms of his hands, and ſoles of his feet, were diſagreeably hot; he was very giddy, quite languid, and had no appetite. His medicine vomited and purged him too, which was the antimonial draught, ſaline mixture and eff antimon.

5th. A ſevere paroxyſm, with a bilious vomiting and purging, came on at midnight, the former of which continued all the night. I ordered him the following draught every two hours, with water and a toaſt for drink: R. tinct. cort. peruv. Huxham. ʒiii. tinct. thebaic. gt. xii. aq. ſimp. ℥iſs, ſacch. alb. ad gratum ſaporem. 6th. He had a tolerable night, and was much eaſier a. m. though quite feeble and dejected. I ordered him a drachm of the cortex every hour; and as his ſtomach would not retain it, I added tinct. theb. gt. x. to each doſe, it agreed very indifferently with him.

7th. He was pretty eaſy all night; but had cold ſweats over him, and his pulſe was ſmall and very irregular. I ordered him a drachm of the cortex every hour, in the form of an electuary; and tinct. cort. peruv. Hux. ʒii. aq. ſimp. ℥i. ſacch. alb. q. ſ. after every doſe, to waſh it down, which agreed tolerably with him, having pukea it ſeldom. 8th. He had an indifferent night, and was no way better. I gave him the medicine, as preſcribed the 5th p. m. His medicine run off by ſtool, and he complained of nothing, although he was evidently worſe.

9th. He reſted better than uſual, his medicine having been continued all night, and a. m. he was hungry and eat a little thin ſago with wine now and then. I ordered him a drachm and a half of the bark every hour, with red port and water, which agreed very well with him, and ſtopped the purging. His pulſe was much firmer.

10th. He reſted well, and a. m. only complained of weakneſs. His bark was continued, as on the 9th, and he had no relapſe. He continued taking the bark, until the 29th of March, when he returned to his duty quite well; the number of doſes, ana ʒi. was gradually diminiſhed in the day, as he acquired

quired ſtrength. The method of treatment in the preceding caſe, is an exception to the general one.

CASE V.

William Turner, ſeaman, aged about 34, who came from a merchant ſhip at Sierra Leon, was ſeized on the 29th February, at 2 p. m. latitude at noon 06° 40″ N. with a chillineſs and headach. At 6 p. m. when he complained his headach was violent, his eyes watered much, and he had a ſevere pain in his right ſide. As he was a ſtrong man and his pulſe full, I ordered ſix ounces of blood to be taken away, which he bore ill---and an antimonial draught with ſubacid drink at night, to be repeated every three hours during the paroxyſm.

2d. At 5 a. m. the paroxyſm abated; but his headach, and pain of his ſide continued, with thirſt and ſickneſs at ſtomach. I preſcribed an emetick for him, which operated well, and procured him two copious ſtools; and gave him his draught at night.

3d. At 2 a. m. a paroxyſm returned with increaſed violence, the pain of his ſide extending to his leg, his pulſe was quick and full, his tongue was white, his thirſt inſatiable, and he raved much. About 5 p. m. there was a ſlight remiſſion, his complaints being very little alleviated. I ordered tart. emet. gr. ſs. tinct. theb. gt. xv. miſt. ſalin. ℥i. m. every three hours, and the pediluvium during the paroxyſm.

4th. He reſted very ill from the pain of his ſide; a difficulty of breathing, and univerſal uneaſineſs. He was coſtive too, and the abdomen tumid. I ordered him ſal. cath. amar. ʒi. diſſolved in a little thin gruel, and to be repeated every hour, until he had ſeveral copious ſtools, which relieved him much. At night he took his draught as uſual.

5th. He had a very reſtleſs night, from a bilious vomiting and purging. I preſcribed the tinct. cort. peruv. and tinct. theb. as in the preceding caſe, with water and toaſt for his drink. 6th. About eleven in the night, a violent exacerbation came on with great inquietude; much pain and oppreſſion about the præcordia, a ſhort frequent cough, a wheezing and laborious breathing, and wild notions and dreams; and all his former complaint , except the vomiting and purging, were greatly increaſed: The pediluvium was repeated, a bliſter applied between his ſhoulders, and camphor. gr. v. with his antimonial medicine, and drink was adminiſtered every three hours.

7th. He was much eaſier, tho his ſpirits and ſtrength were much exhauſted; he was very thirſty, and complained of a burning heat in the palms of his hands, and ſoles of his feet. I ordered him a drachm of the cortex every

every hour, which ſat eaſy on his ſtomach, until a paroxyſm returned p. m. nevertheleſs it was continued.

8th. He reached with his bark ſeveral times in the night. I ordered tinct. theb. gt. x. to be added to every doſe, which kept it on his ſtomach. From 4 to 10 p. m. he had a paroxyſm, during which the bark was continued.

9th. The prickly heat broke out on him, and he found himſelf hungry. I ordered him the bark alone, which agreed very well with him, and a little ſago with wine now and then as he choſe it. He had no return of his fever again: he continued taking bark, until he returned to duty on the 29th of March.

C A S E VI.

M. S. aged about 30, who had never been in a hot climate before, after drooping ſome days, and having been much afraid of ſickneſs from lying aſhore at Sierra Leon, was took at m. on the 2d of March, latitude obſerved 05° 40″ with a chillineſs and reaching that continued ſome hours, and was ſucceeded by great heat, a ſevere headach, pain in his loins, laſſitude, deſpondencey, a fluſhing of his countenance, and thirſt. His pulſe was very quick, though rather ſofter than natural. It being late when he complained, I only ordered the common antimonial draught every two hours, and acidulated drink. 1ſt day, His fever remitted a little in the night; yet he complained of great proſtration of ſtrength, giddineſs and dejection. I ordered him an emetick, which operated very well both by vomit and ſtool. At 10 p. m. a paroxſym came on with increaſed violence, the headach and a pain over his eyes, which were much inflamed, and at the bottoms of the orbits very ſevere; and the lumbago reached quite round the abdomen. I preſcribed the antimonial medicine, as when he firſt complained, with his drink.

2d. He had a very reſtleſs night from a purging; univerſal uneaſineſs and pains, eſpecially in his head and loins; an inſatiable thirſt, and a very dry hot ſkin, together with his other complaints. At 6 p. m. he fell aſleep, which did not at all relieve him, being much diſturbed with frightful dreams. I ordered his medicine to be continued, and the pediluvii.

3d. He had an exceeding bad night, from great deſpondency, wild notions, and a delirium. I ordered him a drachm of the bark every hour, which he puked frequently. I gave him the bark with the ſaline mixture, in a ſtate of efferveſcence. At 10 p. m. when he complained of no pain, tho' his fever continued, his body was open. 4th. His ſkin was hot and dry, and he was troubled much with inquietude and thirſt all night. A. m. he complained of no pain, sighed heavily from great oppression about the scrobiculum cordis, and his pulse was very irregular. At 8 a. m. an exacerbation returned with less violence, which continued until 10 p. m. In its height, I ordered the antimonial medicine every two hours and the pediluvium; and at other times his bark, and a small glass of wine after every dose, which kept it on his stomach very well. The urine that he made during the paroxysm, contained neither cloud nor sediment

5th. He had an uneasy night, and a prickly heat like eruption appeared on his face, breast, and shoulders. A. m. he was much better, I ordered his bark and wine as before, which he only puked twice. At 8 p. m. a slight paroxysm to what the former ones were, came on, and an angry eruption broke out about his mouth. He still continued his bark and wine.

6th. He rested well in the night, and complained only of great weakness and lowness of spirits. I prescribed his bark with wine every hour, as before. He had no return of his fever, and continued to take his bark until the 27th of the month, when he returned quite well to his duty.

CASE VII.

John Willis, marine, aged about 28, a strong man, subject to maniacal complaints, who never had been in a hot climate before, on the evening of the 6th of March, latitude at m. 04° 16″ N. was seized with rigours, and universal pains, but did not complain until a. m. following when his head ached violently, his eyes were greatly inflamed, and his pulse was much oppressed. I ordered twelve onuces of blood to be taken from him; upon weighing it afterwards, I found a pound had been taken away; an emetick in four hours after, which puked him well; an antimonial draught, with plenty of acidulated drink at night; and the pediluvium to be used. The blood was sizy, the serum red and little in quantity, and the crassamentum rather loose.

2d Day his headach and pains still continued. I prescribed a dose of salts, and after their operation was over, the antimonial medicine with the pediluvium and his drink. P. m. his headach remitted a little; he complained of a pain in his breast, and thirst; and his pulse was rather quick and softer than natural.

3d. He had a restless night from an exacerbation of his fever and complaints. A. m. the headach was very troublesome, with a cough, a soreness of his throat, and the pain of his breast. I applied a large blister between his shoulders, and continued his medicines as before. 4th. He rested indifferently, though the fever was moderate all night; and complained still of his headach, universal pains, and thirst. His antimonial medicine was repeated every four hours.

hours. 5th. There was no alteration for the better, and he was very coſtive. ℞. cath. amar. ſal. pulv. cort. peruv a ℥vi. ſucc. til. mar. fruct. ℥ii. pulmenttarii lb. ſs. m. quadran. Æger unaquaque hora ſumat. His medicine purged him only once; he was very cool at night. 6th. He was much better, and took his bark as before. 7th. The bark was preſcribed with elix. vitr. and he continued taking it, only diminiſhing the number of doſes daily, until the 17th of the month, when he returned to duty quite well. Three other marines, who were of the watering party too at Sierra Leon, had the ſame fever, and recovered by the ſame means in twenty five days the worſt of them.

CASE VIII.——*St. Thomas's Fever.*

William Lauchlan, ſeaman, aged about 50, on the 24th of April 1772,* p. m. was ſeized with a chillineſs, headach, and ſevere univerſal pains. Next morning when he complained after having been very hot, thirſty, and reſtleſs through the night, his ſkin was dry and hot, his pulſe quick, his tongue whiteiſh, his thirſt inſatiable, and he found his ſtrength and ſpirits proſtrated. I ordered him an emetick, which operated well; and the antimonial mixture every four hours, with nitre in his drink. At 9 p. m. there was a ſmall remiſſion.

2d. He reſted very ill in the night, he was very weak, giddy, his thirſt irreſiſtable, and his pulſe quick and ſmall. I preſcribed a doſe of ſalts for him, and his draught at night, with his drink. At 6 p. m an exacerbation came on, which remitted a little at 10 p. m. 3d. He had no reſt in the night, a violent paroxyſm having come on at 1 a. m. with a frequent cough, and great deſpondency, beſides his former complaints. His tongue was foul too, and he was coſtive. A 3 p. m there was a ſmall remiſſion, during which the ſymptoms and thirſt were ſcarcely alleviated. I continued his medicine every two hours in the paroxyſm, and every four in the remiſſion. Another exacerbation with a dyſuria began at 9 p. m.

4th. He was quite languid from great inquietude in the night. There was a ſmall remiſſion at 6 a. m. tho' his head was like to ſplit; the univerſal pains were ſevere, particularly in his loins; the palms of his hands and ſoles of his feet were very hot, and his thirſt continued. I preſcribed ſal. cath. amar. ℥ſs. which gave him ſeveral ſtoo s; afterwards repeated the antimonial medicine, and made him uſe the pediluvium.

5th. His cough was very troubleſome, which increaſed his headach, and his pulſe was very irregular. At 4 p. m. an exacerbation of the fever and ſymptoms

* Latitude at noon 00° 09″ Sout

ſymptoms returned with great pain about the ſcrobiculum cordis, and remitted imperfectly at 6. At 8 p. m. it increaſed again with greater violence, and his tongue was brown and rough.

6th. There was a ſmall remiſſion at 11 in the night; and at 12 a violent paroxyſm came on. Beſides his former complaints, which were greatly increaſed, he had a great pain about his throat, over his eyes, and at the bottoms of the orbits; when he coughed, his eyes were like to fly out of his head, and he raved much. At 4 a. m. there was a ſlight remiſſion; at 6 the paroxyſm returned, and remitted again imperfectly at 4 p. m. His pulſe was very irregular, and a diſagreeable ſenſation remained on the fingers for ſome time after feeling it—as indeed happened in every caſe. I applied a large bliſter between his ſhoulders; repeated his medicine with pulv. contrayerv. c. camphor. ana gr. vi. made into a bolus, every three hours. 7th. He was in leſs pain in the night, tho' his cough continued inceſſant, and he was quite languid. I ordered him a drachm of the bark, with a little wine every hour; and though he puked it ſeveral times, he was rather eaſier at night.

8th. He complained chiefly of his cough. He continued his bark and wine, which agreed very well with him and at night he was cool, and his cough leſs. Laſt twenty-four hours he took two ounces and a half of bark.

9th. He continued taking his medicine in the night, and had no complaint but of weakneſs. I ordered the bark every two hours, only with wine, of which he had his allowance. He afterwards took it with elix. vitr. until the 8th of May, when he returned to duty. I gave him the decoction with elix. vitr. for ſome time after. This was one of the caſes who relapſed with the change of weather.

CASE IX.

Peter Williams, ſeaman, a very ſtrong molattoe creole, aged about 34, on the 27th of April, latitude at m. 00° 41 ſ. at 10 a. m. was ſeized with ſevere rigours, which continued two hours; a violent headach, ſickneſs at ſtomach, univerſal pains, eſpecially in his loins, and an ardent fever, with vehement thirſt. Great anxiety ſucceeded, which terminated in a very profuſe ſweat. As he did not complain until it was late in the evening, I only ordered him the antimonial mixture and ſubacid drink.

1ſt. About midnight there was a degree of remiſſion. A. m. I ordered him an emetick: in two hours after its operation was over, ſal. cath. amar. ℥i, and at night the antimonial medicine to be repeated every four hours, with ſubacid drink. 2d. At 11 in the night, the fever and ſymptoms came on with greater violence, and a delirium, it remitted a little at 4 a. m. it returned

again

again at 10 a. m. with chillinefs, and continued fevere until 8 p. m. Together with his former complaints, he had great pain and ftricture about his eyes, which were much inflamed, and he was coftive. During the imperfect remiffions, there was a great proftration of his ftrength and fpirits, with giddinefs; he had univerfal pains and uneafinefs, and his thirft was infatiable. I repeated the antimonial medicine every two hours in the paroxyfms, with his drink, and made him ufe the pediluvium.

3d. He had a better night. I ordered him fal. cath. amar. ʒvi. with thin gruel, which procured him feveral copious ftools; and his antimonial medicine and drink at night. At 6 p. m. an exacerbation with increafed violence commenced, together with the former fymptoms, which were all more violent; he had a bilious vomiting and purging, a dyfuria, and great inquietude.

4th. He was very much difturbed with the delirium, inquietude, and vomiting and purging all night. At 7 a. m. there was a flight remiffion, during which his pulfe was full and very foft; his tongue was remarkably fmooth, he was greatly dejected, quite languid, had a bitter tafte in his mouth, and a burning heat in his palms and foles. I prefcribed the antimonial medicine in an effervefcent ftate, with tinct. thebaic. applied a large blifter between his fhoulders, and repeated the pediluvium. At 6 p. m a paroxyfm began, during which he raved greatly, and was comatofe. I ordered pulv. contrayerv. c. camphor. ana gr. vi. quartaquaque hora, with his other medicines.

5th. At 10 in the night, there was a flight remiffion, which continued two hours only. A moft violent paroxyfm commenced then with great oppreffion about the fcrobiculum cordis. He was highly delirious and outrageous with extreme watching; his tongue was black, and his other complaints were much more fevere, except the coma. About 7 a. m. there was a very imperfect remiffion; I continued his medicines during the paroxyfm, as prefcribed the preceding day, and applied blifters to his ankles. At 7 a. m. I ordered him cort. peruv. pulv. ʒifs. every hour, with a little wine; and at 10 p. m. he found himfelf eafy and cool, having taken twenty-two drachms of the bark, which agreed with him.

6th. Between 12 and 2 a. m. he had a very flight paroxyfm; at other times was quiet and eafy, and took his medicine. P. m. he was very eafy all day, having took a drachm of the bark every hour, with a little elix. vitr. and I allowed him his wine. 7th. He had a good night's reft, and was recovering. I prefcribed the bark with elix. vitr. every two hours, and gave him his wine.

8th. He continued to recover, and took half an ounce of bark. Afterwards he had the decoction with elix. vitr. and would return to his duty the 7th of May. The change of the weather affected him frequently afterwards.

CASE X.

James Ayſlop, aged about 15, of a very thin and paralytick habit, who never had been in a hot climate before, was taken ill at the ſame time as the preceding caſe, with the general ſymptoms; and when he complained next morning, he was worſe in every reſpect, after a reſtleſs night. I ordered him an emetick; and in two hours after its operation. ſal. cath. amar. ℥i. with thin gruel. At noon a remiſſion began, and at night I gave him the antimonial medicine, with ſubacid drink.

2d day. He had a tolerable night, but complained of great weakneſs, giddineſs, and that his medicine griped him. To every doſe thereof, which he took every four hours, I added a few drops of tinct. thebaic. At 4 p. m. a ſevere exacerbation came on, and remitted imperfectly at 10, during which he had ſeveral bilious ſtools.

3d. At midnight a paroxyſm returned, which remitted at 6 a. m. and left him quite languid and dejected, together with the uſual complaints. At 4 p. m. another exacerbation began and remitted a little at 8. As he was coſtive, the antimonial medicine was given in ſmall quantities every two hours, without the tinct. theb. 4th. A ſevere paroxyſm, preceded by griping, commenced at midnight, and remitted at 7 a. m. all his complaints were more troubleſome, and he continued to take his medicine. 5th. He was tolerable eaſy in the night, but had no ſleep. At 6 p. m. an exacerbation came on, which continued only a few hours: the remiſſion was very imperfect, and his medicine was preſcribed as before.

6th. His complaints all continued, and he was in no reſpect better. I ordered him a drachm of the bark every hour; through negligence, he only had been given one or two doſes—P. m. he was reather weaker. 7th. His tongue was very foul, and the other ſymptoms were very troubleſome in the night; yet he took his bark every hour, and continued it all day, with a little wine to every doſe, which agreed very well with him.

8th. He was much better, and complained of weakneſs only. I preſcribed his bark as before, which he continued to take—only diminiſhing the number of doſes, until the 10th of May, when he returned to his duty. He took the decoction with elix. vitr. twice a day, for ſome time after.

CASE XI.

Thomas Dale, marine, aged about 38, who never had been in a hot climate before, on the 30th of April, at 8 p. m. latitude obſerved 02° 10 S. was

was ſeized with all the general ſymptoms; and at midnight, they and the fever remitted for a little only. Next day at m. when I ſaw him, all his complaints were much ſeverer, with deafneſs. I ordered him an emetick, which operated well; and the antimonial draught at night, with nitre in his drink. P. M. a ſmall remiſſion appeared.

2d. He reſted very ill, being troubled with much inquietude, and the lumbago. I preſcribed an ounce of the ſal. cath. amar. with thin gruel, and the uſual medicine at night. 3 P. m. he complained of being very chilly, though his ſkin was hot and dry, and his pulſe was quick.

3d. He had a very reſtleſs night, and no remiſſion appeared until 8 p. m. All the ſymptoms were increaſed in violence, in the paroxyſm, and it left him quite languid and deſponding. With the ſaline mixture, I ordered him tart. emet. gr. ſs. every four hours, and ſubacid drink.

4th. He had a very indifferent night; he was very giddy, languid, and thirſty, with the uſual complaints; and nothing pleaſed his taſte. I ordered him the antimonial mixture as before. 5th. An exacerbation returned at 10 in the night, and continued until 7 p. m. with an urgent cough, and pain about the ſcrobiculum cordis. I preſcribed for him as on the third. 6th. He reſted ill, and was greatly dejected. I ordered him a drachm of the cortex, with a little wine every hour. At 6 p. m. a paroxyſm began, in the height of which he took the antimonial mixture.

7th. Early a. m. there was a remiſſion, and he took his bark and wine every hour, which agreed very well with him. Though his paroxyſms were not violent, he was nevertheleſs much weaker than others who had more ſevere ones. 8th. He was recovering, and continued to take his bark as before.

9th. He had a ſlight paroxyſm in the night. I ordered the elix. vitr. with his bark every hour, and allowed him his wine. 10th, 11th, and 12th, I gave him half an ounce of bark daily; and afterwards the decoction twice a day, with the elix. vitr. which he continued to take for ſome time after he returned to duty, on the 15th of May.

C A S E XII.

Henry Annas, ſeaman, a ſtrong man, aged about 37, on the evening of the 29th of April, lat. obſerved 01° 45″ S. was ſuddenly ſeized with giddineſs and faintneſs, which were followed with a violent headach, an acute pain of his loins, and univerſal pains, and heat, with great thirſt. When he complained on the firſt of May, all his com laints were more ſevere; he was ſick at his ſtomach, and his pulſe was ſtrong and quick. I ordered him an emetick, the antimonial draugh s every four hours after, ſubacid drink and the

the pediluvium to be ufed In the evening there was an imperfect remiffion, only for the firft time.

2d day. At 1 a. m. a paroxyfm began with rigours, which continued until 6 p. m. when he complained of great proftration of ftrength and univerfal forenefs; his thirft was infatiable, and his pulfe foft, befides the general complaints of dejection, burning heat in the palms of his hands, and the foles of his feet; a bitter tafte in his mouth, and nothing pleafed his tafte. I ordered him an ounce of fal. cath. amar. and after they were wrought off, the fame medicines as the preceding night, with plenty of drink. At 9 p. m. an exacerbation of the fever and fymptoms commenced.

3d. He was troubled with great inquietude, and the fever continued until 1 a. m. when he was feized with rigours which lafted three hours, and a moft violent paroxyfm followed, that continued until 4 p. m. His former complaints were greatly exacerbated; and he had a dyfuria; a great pain and ftricture about his eyes; an oppreffion about the fcrobiculum cordis; his tongue was brown and dry, and his mouth parched, and he wandered at times. In the remiffion, his fpirits and ftrength were quite proftrated, and he was very giddy. I continued the antimonial medicine, in the Sp. Minder. with fubacid drink, and the pediluvium every two hours in the paroxyfm—His body was fufficiently open.

4th. He had a tolerable night; and early a. m. another acceffion of the fever and fymptoms began, and continued until 4 p. m. but were not fo violent as on the preceding day. His medicines were repeated as before.

5th. He was eafy in the night. At 2 p. m. he was fuddenly taken fpeechlefs; and fome time after I was fent for to fee him, and was told he was juft dying. When I faw him, he lay on his back, his eyes were not quite clofed, his countenance was very ghaftly, and covered with a cold clammy fweat, as was his breaft; his extremities were cold, his hands were folded over the fcrobiculum cordis; his pulfe was thready, tremulous, and vermicular at times; the hypochondria were tumid; he was wholly fenfelefs and motionlefs, excepting convulfive twiches about his mouth. He continued in this lifelefs ftate about an hour, notwithftanding he was well rubbed with flannel clothes fprinkled with volatiles, without altering his pofture; as foon as he could fwallow, fome drops were given him internally, with a little drink; and when the tibiæ internæ were well rubbed in that manner, they were embrocated with warm vinegar, and large blifters applied to them. After that apoplexy, fyncope, or whatever any one choofes to call it, a mere frenzy followed. His countenance was exceedingly flufhed, his eyes were greatly inflamed, the mufcles of the neck were quite rigid, the abdomen tenfe, his fkin burning hot, his pulfe was very irregular, with a fubfultus tendinum; he was highly delirious and unmanageable, and his tongue quite black and dry. I covered his

his back with a bliſter, adminiſtered pulv. contrayerv. c. & camphor. ana gr. viii. twice, and his antimonial medicine was repeated every hour, with plenty of ſubacid drink before 9 p. m. when the ſweat began. I then preſcribed two drachms of the cortex, with wine and a little tinct. theb. every hour, which his ſtomach retained.

6th. His medicine was given him regularly all night, though there was no ſign of a remiſſion until midnight, and he continued taking his bark after the ſame manner until 4 p. m. when a paroxyſm returned, which was as ſlight as the preceding remiſſion was moderate and dinſtinct. From the time that he began to take the bark, until the return of the paroxyſm which was nineteen hours, he ſwallowed and kept down four ounces and an half of bark. He then took only a drachm for a doſe.

7th. At midnight he became quite cool, and continued his bark and wine.

8th. He was recovering, tho' very weak, and took his bark regularly every hour.

9th. The bark was preſcribed with elixir of vitriol every hour, and his wine allowed him. Before the 15th, when he would return to his duty, he had taken a pound of the bark in powder; and for ſome time after, I gave him twice a day, an infuſion of it in wine. He was very ſlightly affected with the change of weather afterwards.

A number more of our men had the fever, from lying aſhore at St. Thomas's, but all recovered from the ſame method of treatment.

Caſes of the Remitting Fever on the Second Voyage.

C A S E XIII.

William Peer, marine, aged about 26, who never was in a hot climate before, on the 30th of March 1773, latitude obſerved 05° 29″ N. was ſeized with a pain and oppreſſion about the pit of the ſtomach an inclination to vomit and giddineſs. I ordered him an emetick, the antimonial medicine at night, and ſubacid drink.

2d day. Though he ſweated profuſely in the night, and his ſkin was much cooler a. m. all his complaints continued. I preſcribed an ounce of ſalts for him; and his mixture with drink at night. 3d. He had a very bad night, and at 4 a. m. a ſevere exacerbation, preceded by rigours, came on, attended with a bilious vomiting and griping, a heavineſs of his head, a great pain in his loins, a proſtration of his ſtrength and ſpirits, a very quick ſmall pulſe, an urgent thirſt, and an increaſed violence of his other complaints; towards night it remitted, and left him quite languid and dejected, together with the uſual ſymptoms. As his ſalts did not purge him the preceding day, I gave

 him

him ſal. cath. amar. ℥ii. every hour, in ſome warm thin gruel, until he had ſome ſtools, and afterwards, his antimonial medicine and drink.

4th. He was troubled with much inquietude in the night. At 2 a. m. an acceſſion of his fever came on, and remitted at 7, during which he had four copious ſtools. He took his medicine every four hours. P. m. he was eaſier, tho very weak, and his tongue foul, with a bad taſte in his mouth.

5th. At 2 a. m. a paroxyſm with an increaſed violence of his former complaints, returned. He vomited ſeverely, and felt great pain upon preſſing the pit of the ſtomach. There was an imperfect remiſſion at 8. An exacerbation came on again at 11 a. m. which remitted at 6 p. m. when he complained of coſtiveneſs, giddineſs, proſtration of his ſtrength, and very great deſpondency. I continued his medicine and drink.

6th. He had an eaſier night. I ordered him a drachm and an half of bark, with two drachms of ſal. cath. amar. and repeated his bark every hour, with a little wine, which agreed with him, and he had ſeveral ſtools.

7th. He had a good night, was free of fever, complained of weakneſs only; and took eighteen drachms of bark, with wine and water. He continued to take his bark until the 13th of April, only decreaſing the number of doſes daily, when he returned to his duty. I gave him twice a day for ſome time after, a wine infuſion of the bark.

C A S E XIV.

Francis Eaſtmond, marine, a ſtrong man, on the 9th of April 1773— Latitude obſerved, 04° 23″ N. a. m. was ſeized with rigours, which were followed by the general complaints, and in the evening there was an imperfect remiſſion of them. I ordered him an emetick, the antimonial medicine at night, and nitre in his drink.

2d. About 10 in the night, an exacerbation came on; he was much troubled with inquietude, and had a great pain and ſtricture over his eyes, and at the bottom of his orbits, with all his former complaints. At 6 p. m. there was a ſlight remiſſion only. I gave him ſal. cath. amar. ℥i. and at night repeated his medicine every four hours, with his drink.

3d. He had an indifferent night, and at 6 a. m. a paroxyſm commenced with rigours; and, together with his former complaints, was attended with an irregular pulſe, a foul tongue, watching, and a delirium. I applied a large bliſter between his ſhoulders, ordered him camphor. gr. viii. which he nauſeated, and the ſp. minder. with eſſ. ant. every four hours, and made his feet and legs be put in warm water.

4th. His fever remitted at 7 a. m. but he was very coſtive. I repeated the doſe of ſalts, which gave him ſeveral copious ſtools; and afterwards his antimonial

timonial mixture as before. A very angry eruption broke out about his mouth and nofe.

5th. At 4 a. m. an exacerbation returned again with rigours; a bilious vomiting, and an immoderate difcharge of urine, befides the other fymptoms, which remitted at m. I ordered him his antimonial medicine every two hours, and repeated the pediluvium.

6th. He was extremely weak, giddy and dejected. I ordered him a drachm of the bark every hour, and allowed him wine. 7th. He was recovering, and continued his medicines. He took the bark in fubftance, until the 18th of the month, when he returned to duty, and afterwards an infufion of it in wine, twice a day.

Cafes which occurred during the laft Voyage.

CASE XV.

The following cafe properly fpeaking, is anomalous, becaufe three feparate and very different fevers happened therein—namely, a catarrhous, a hectick, and a remittent—but as it is not only an uncommon one, but terminated in a putrid remittent, I fhall infert it here under the prefent head at full length.

Richard Spurret, marine, aged about 36, on the 20th of December 1773, latitude obferved, 25° 02″ complained of a pain and fwelling in the left fide of his face, that had feized him in the night; he was thirfty, and his pulfe was quick and hard. I ordered a few ounces of blood to be taken from him; effen, antimon. gt. xxx. to be given him at night, with acidulated fage tea; and a volatile liniment fprinkled on a piece of flannel, to be applied to his face.

21ft. His face was eafier, the epithem was renewed; abftinence from falt provifions enjoined, and the eff. antimon. with the fage tea, was repeated at night. 22d. His face and fame fide of his throat were much fwelled; he had a pain in fwallowing, coughed at times, and his pulfe was quick, though not hard. I prefcribed a dofe of fal. cath. amar. and a gargarifm of fage tea, diftilled vinegar and honey, to be made ufe of frequently; a bolus of fperm. cet. and nitre at night, and the epithem to be continued.

23d. The fwelling was more enlarged and harder, his pulfe was ftill quick and his fkin dryer and hotter than in health. I ordered a fomentation and the epthem to be renewed twice a day; I repeated his bolus morning and evening; and at night gave him the eff. antimon. with his drink. He was fubject to a cough and complaints in his breaft.

24th.

24th. The parotis was lefs, he had no pain in it, and deglutition was eafy but his tongue was foul, his cough without any expectoration was more urgent, which occafioned his head to ach; and he complained of a pain in his back. His body was open. I gave him a linctus of fperm. cet. mel. brit. & oxymel. fcill. with a few drops of fp. vitr. ten. to take the fize of a nutmeg of when the cough was moft urgent; I continued his other medicines, ordered him an opiate at night, and the pediluvium.

25th. He found himfelf much better, and coughed lefs. I ordered all his medicines to be continued. 26th. He got cold, and coughed all night, which raifed his headach again and a great pain in his breaft, that made refpiration difficult. His pulfe was now quick and fuller than in health. I made a few ounces of blood be taken from him, gave him acidulated ptifan for his common drink, and continued his other medicines.

27th. The fwelling and pain had entirely left his face and throat; he had a pain and oppreffion about the pit of his ftomach, a watching and colliquative fweats. P. m. his complaints were more fevere he raved, and his pulfe was fmall, quick, and hard. I applied a large blifter to his back; inftead of the linctus I gave him the lack ammoniac. with oxymel. fcil & eff. antimon. and continued his drink. P. m. I opened both the venæ faphenæ, after ufing the pediluvium; added tinct. theb. gt. v. to every dofe of his mixture, and allowed the common emulfion with nitre, and the ptifan for his drink.

28th. He was in great pain about the thorax, breathed with difficulty, was extremely reftlefs and delirious the firft part of the night; towards morning he grew better, expectorated a little, had two copious ftools, and I continued his medicines.

29th. He refted well, coughed little, expectorated more, breathed eafy, and had no fever. He took his mixture every four hours, continued his drink, and had an opiate at night only. 30th. He was much better, and his medicines were repeated.

31ft. He had a ftraitnefs about the thorax, efpecially the right fide, and coughed frequently. I repeated his medicines and drink, ordered him to ufe the pediluvium, and applied a large blifter to the affected fide.

January 1ft, 1774. He refted well, expectorated eafily, though he was breathlefs from walking up or down the ladder, and complained of his blifters paining him much. I continued his medicines. 2d. From his opiate having been neglected, he coughed, and was reftlefs until he got it; he was eafy in the day; he made ufe of his former linctus, with ptifan, and had his opiate at night.

3d. He had no cough in the night, and complained of a weaknefs in his loins only. His medicine was continued, and the bliftered parts kept open.

The

The colliquative ſweats were not gone. 4th. There was no alteration on him. Beſides continuing his linctus, I ordered him a drachm of the bark, with elix. vitr. four times a day.

5th. His cough was troubleſome in the night. I ordered him the bark only twice a day; and as he was feveriſh, I gave him camphor. gr. v. quatuor in die, and continued his linctus, ptiſan, and opiate. 6th. He had a quieter night, yet the colliquative ſweats weakened him exceedingly. P. m. he had chills and heats alternately. I omitted the camphor, and preſcribed half an ounce of bark, to be taken with elix. vitr. and continued his other medicines and drink.

7th. He was extremely weak from the ſweats; he had a ſmall fever conſtantly, and a headach, from a continual irritating cough. Inſtead of the linctus, I ordered him ol. olivar. opt. ʒi. now and then; his anodyne at night, the emulſion and ptiſan for drink, and his bark which made him ſick p. m. 8th. He had a purging in the night, which relieved him a little. I repeated his anodyne twice, and continued his other medicines.

9th. He reſted tolerably in the night, and his body kept open; though the fever continued, and his breathing was laborious, he complained of no pain. P. m. His ſtomach and abdomen were much puffed up, and he was very deſirous to break wind. Towards night he became very reſtleſs; he was faintiſh at times, his countenance was wild, and he raved. I omitted the bark, adminiſtered an emollient injection, renewed the bliſter on his ſide, gave him equal parts of wine and water frequently, and the emulſion with nitre for his drink, The injection procured him ſeveral ſtools and a free diſcharge of wind, which relieved him.

10th. He was very reſtleſs, and ſweated profuſely at every pore until morning, and the cough was ſtill very urgent. I continued the wine, with a very light diet, and gave him an anodyne at night. 11th. He ſweated leſs, was extremely weak, his pulſe was very ſmall, his tongue was rough and white in the middle, a tickling in his throat brought on the cough, he expectorated a little phlegm only, and was coſtive. I ordered the injection to be repeated, which gave him two copious ſtools; his medicines and diet, as on the preceding day, to be continued, and gave him a ſoft linctus to lick at pleaſure.

12th. He reſted well, coughed little, and expectorated eaſily; his pulſe was regular, he was cool, had little thirſt, and an appetite, but was ſtill coſtive. I continued all his medicines.

13th. He had very little cough, and complained only of great weakneſs, and of being coſtive. I ordered him two ounces of a decoction of ſena, tamarinds, and cardamom. min. which gave him three copious ſtools. P. m. he had a little cough, and his medicines were repeated.

14th. He complained only of weaknefs. I prefcribed a drachm of the bark twice a day, with wine and the elix. vitr. which agreed with him. 15th. He continued better, and took his bark as before, with a nourifhing diet.

16th. He complained of being coftive. I gave him fal. cath. amar. ℥ii. which made him cough and fpit up fome phlegm. Afterwards, he took his bark at four dofes, inftead of two, with his wine as before. 17th. He did not recover any ftrength. I increafed his bark to half an ounce a day, which he tock as before.

Now commenced his Remitting Fever.

18th. He had no cough, but was very hot, the firft part of the night, and perfpired freely after. I continued his bark, wine, and diet. At 6 p. m. he was feized with a chillinefs, which was fucceeded by a fever, hæmorrhage at the nofe, and thirft that went off by a profufe perfpiration. During the paroxyfm, I prefcribed the fp. minderer. and fage tea.

19th. He was quite weak, efpecially in his loins, and thirfty. I ordered him a drachm of the bark with wine every hour. At 3 p. m. a fevere exacerbation of the fever, with the hæmorrhage, a violent headach, great pain in his loins, a purging, and urgent thirft, came on. The fp. minderer. and tinct. theb. were prefcribed, together with his drink.

20th. The paroxyfm continued, the hæmorrhage returned in the night, and he complained of great pain in his knees. At 5 p. m. he was feized with chillinefs, and a reaching, which were followed by the fever, hæmorrhage and other complaints. I added tinct. theb. gt. x. to the dofe of bark, which I gave him every hour, together with his wine.

21ft. Without any remiffion, another exacerbation of his fever came on in the night, with a very profufe hæmorrhage, at leaft to the quantity of ℔. iv. before it was ftopped with doffils immerfed in the tinct. ftypt. plugged up his nofe, and opiates adminiftered internally. His extremities then were cold, his pulfe was vermicular, he was covered with a cold fweat, his countenance was ghaftly, and he was quite faint. At 7 a. m a paroxyfm returned with rigours, and a puking, which was troublefome through the day. His extremities were frequently well rubbed with flannel clothes fprinkled with volatiles, and then wrapped in them; the bark with wine and tinct. theb. was regularly repeated every hour, and at intervals I ordered him a little wine. P m. his extremities became warm; an equable and moderate perfpiration broke out over him, and he was in tolerable pirits.

22d. He was reftlefs and puked once the firft part of the night. His medicine agreed with him, and he flept a little towards morning. His pulfe was much firmer, he was quite cool, and complained of weaknefs only. I continued

tinued his medicines, and allowed him wine, and mutton broth now and then, off which all the fat was carefully ſcummed.

23d. He reſted well, and had no fever or any complaint, only of weakneſs. I preſcribed the bark, a drachm every hour as before, with wine only, which agreed very well with him, and his diet as on the preceding day.

24th. He had regular ſtools, without any particular complaint, except of low ſpiritedneſs. I continued his bark, wine, and diet. His medicine, wine, and a nouriſhing diet were regularly adminiſtered, and no alteration happened until the 2d of February, when he complained of his feet and legs ſwelling towards night otherwiſe he was much recovered. I ordered him half an ounce of bark daily, his pint of wine and diet.

3d. The prickly heat broke out over him, and he complained only of weakneſs, particularly in his loins, and of his legs being ſwelled at night. No alteration was made in his preſcriptions. 5th. His countenance was rather bloated, though he was greatly recovered. I ordered him a wine infuſion of the bark, with elix. vitr. twice a day, which he continued for a conſiderable time, although he returned to ſentinels duty on the 8th of February.

In June following, he was ſeized with ſcorbutick ſymptoms, and complained much at times, of the weakneſs and pain of his loins, of which he recovered, and came home in good health.

This man took above a pound of the bark in powder; what he uſed in the infuſion, I am not certain, although I know that the quantity was conſiderable.

CASE XVI.

M. R. aged about 32, of a thin habit, from careleſſly expoſing himſelf to the ſun, and unuſual fatigue on the afternoon of the 16th of June, his perſpiration ſtopped, and he was ſeized with univerſal ſevere wandering pains, great laſſitude, anxiety, and a burning heat in the palms of his hands and ſoles of his feet; his pulſe was full and quick, and his urine which he voided with heat, was high coloured, and in a ſmall quantity. I ordered him the pediluvium, the antimonial medicine, and plenty of acidulated drink. In the evening, all his complaints and thirſt were greatly exacerbated.

17th. He reſted ill from great inquietude; he had ſhort partial ſweats, with an intolerable heat in the palms of his hands and ſoles of his feet; his thirſt was inſatiable, his pulſe was ſtrong and quick, and the temporal arteries throbbed vehemently. A. m. he was a little relieved, though he had a ſevere headach, and his urine, which was leſs in quantity, was darkiſh coloured, and quite turbid. I ordered him of ſal. cath. glaub. mann. ana ℥iſs. which made him vomit a little, and purged him well. P. m. he found himſelf eaſier, yet

none

none of his complaints were entirely removed. I repeated the pediluvium and antimonial medicine with his drink.

18th. He refted better, and his complaints were all more moderate, except the dyfuria, which was more fevere; his urine was very little in quantity, of a very dark colour, thickifh, and was full of bloody fibres, and he found himfelf very giddy when he got out of bed. I repeated his antimonial medicine a. m. and added fp. nitr d to his drink. At 10 a. m. an exacerbation of the fever and his complaints commenced with the headach, and p. m, he was fent to fick quarters.—As I was favoured with an account of the following part of his cafe, I fhall beg leave to infert it.

In the evening he was ordered the pediluvium, the antimonial medicine, and tamarind beverage for his drink, with fp. nitr. dul. in it. His urine then was neither fo dark coloured nor fo thick.

19th. He refted very ill, tho' there was a remiffion of his fever and complaints at midnight. His purge, with the addition of fome of cryft. tart. was repeated, which operated very well. P. m. he found himfelf better, and the dyfuria was abated. The medicines were repeated at night, as before.

20th. His fever was moderate, after a tolerable night's reft; and he voided his urine eafier, in a larger quantity, and clearer, yet his headach was troublefome. He was ordered a drachm of the bark every hour, with water only, and it agreed with him. P. m. his headach remitted at 2 p. m. and though he had taken an ounce of bark, his ufual medicines and drink were prefcribed at night.

21ft. He had no return of his fever; but the pain in voiding his urine did not leave him for a confiderable time, and he continued taking the bark eight days, though after the fourth he diminifhed the quantity daily.

I have now candidly delivered all the remarks, which I have hitherto made on the remitting fever, which happened on board of fhips upon the coaft of Africa, at fuch a diftance from the land, as that neither the exhalations nor the effluvia emitted therefrom, could be fuppofed to have any immediate influence on the fick, except the laft cafe; notwithftanding thefe very caufes gave rife to, or occafioned the fever on board of the Weafel, in the river Gambia, chiefly; on board of the Rainbow, in Sierra Leon river folely, and I may fay, at St. Thomas' likewife.

I have already acknowledged the fimplicity and inelegancy of the manner in which I treated my patients; but the fuccefs that attended it, is a better apology for it, if not a vindication, than words could poffibly exprefs.

I cannot help obferving, that I certainly would have adminiftered the bark earlier, had I not been perfuaded to the contrary, by an eminent phyfician and friend of mine, before I went out in the Rainbow, in a difcourfe which

which we then had upon that head. However, I ſhall with all deference, beg leave to diſſent from the Doctor's opinion in that circumſtance hereafter, as I did indeed in a few caſes; becauſe, I think, to delay giving the bark after the ſtomach and *primæ viæ* are emptied of their contents, eſpecially when there is a remiſſion, is loſing time. Beſides, in the caſes which I adminiſtered on the third day, no unfavourable ſymptoms ever happend in conſequence thereof.

CHAP. II.

OF THE DYSENTERY.

SECTION I.

The Dyſentery deſcribed which happened at Jamaica.

THE general complaints of the dyſenterick patients at Jamaica, were at firſt frequent looſe ſtools, in ſome patients with, and in others without blood or gripes; a ſoreneſs of the belly, as they termed it; a pain and weakneſs of the loins, together with a nauſea and thirſt; the pulſe was quicker, and the ſkin hotter, and dryer than natural.

When the diſeaſe had its own courſe for two, three, or more days before they complained, which was too often the caſe, the account of its beginning and advancement, which I got from them, was very diſtinct, and the ſymptoms varied then according to the manner in which they had lived, and the time that they had been ill.

However, many were ſeized at firſt with a chillineſs or rigours; a reaching, bloody ſtools, violent gripes, a twiſting of their guts, as if they had been cramped or contracted into knots; and as if they had been pierced with knives; for in all theſe different ways they expreſſed themſelves; a teneſmus, a hæmorrhage at the noſe, a numbedneſs of the feet, a great proſtration of the ſtrength and ſpirits, and faintneſs. The more of theſe that there were concurring in one caſe, the more dangerous it always proved.

But in whatever manner they were firſt ſeized, their caſes ſoon became nearly ſimilar, and differed only in degrees of violence, unleſs they were relieved by the firſt evacuations, which I am ſorry to ſay, happened too ſeldom. Their ſtools which at firſt were large, and ſomewhat excrementitious, in ſome caſes with, and in others without blood, as I have already obſerved, and conti-

 nued

nued ſo throughout the diſeaſe, ſoon diminiſhed in quantity, became more frequent, and of a watery, ſlimy, or mucous conſiſtence, mixed or ſtreaked with blood; in ſome caſes they appeared like the *Carnium Lotura,* and in others like mere ſanies: the gripes and teneſmus continued to increaſe daily with very little reſpite, until the diſeaſe either became chronical, or until the ſtrength of the patients was exhauſted, and a mortification took place; when the pain ceaſed, their ſtools ran off involuntarily, and death put an end to their calamity, which was always preceded by one or more black putrid, and very fetid ſtools.

In the courſe of the diſeaſe many more alarming ſymptoms occurred; namely, very hot ſtools *; a procidentia ani; an amazing dilatation in ano *; a profuſe hæmorrhage ab ano *; a dyſuria; a ſuppreſſion of the urine, eſpecially towards night; great tenſion and pain in the abdomen; flatulencies; a ſevere pain about the pubis; a vomiting, particularly after taking any thing; a vomiting of worms; a voracious appetite; aptha; a ſenſe of great internal heat; pain and ſoreneſs of the eyes; a tinnitus aurium; a wildneſs in the countenance; great anxiety and reſtleſſneſs, a delirium, a hiccup, an hippocratick countenance, a deliquium, involuntary ſtools, and a cadaverous ſmell.

Some of the latter may be reckoned ſymptoms of the fever, which differed both in degree of ſtrength and malignancy amongſt them, but kept pace with the flux, and towards night there was generally an exacerbation. The pulſe was ſometimes quick, ſmall, and irregular, and at others very languid, though very often it was not to be depended upon, becauſe of the patient's fatigue from getting frequently out and in to bed: However, it generally ſank gradually, and was either very ſmall, tremulous, or vermicular, with a ſubſultus tendinum before death. The tongue from being white at firſt, became daily more foul, and at length either brown or black, and the teeth cruſted over with ſordes, the thirſt was generally inſatiable, the ſkin moſt commonly in the beginning was hot and dry, but towards the fatal period there were partial and cold clammy ſweats, particularly on the face and breaſt, and the extremities were cold.

SECTION II.

The Difference between the Jamaica *Dyſentery and the one which happened to the Southward of the Equator.*

IN the dyſentery which happened to the Southward of the Equator, the ſickneſs at ſtomach, the gripes, pain in different places, and contortion of the bowels, were more violent, and the proſtration of ſtrength and ſpirits were much

* Theſe ſymptoms have not been taken notice of by any author which I have read.

much greater. Befides, fome were attacked with alternate rigours and heats, voilent headaches and vomitings, and very quick and full pulfes. Others were at once feized with frequent purgings of blood, and violent gripes without a feverifh fymptom. In one cafe that proved fatal the third day, a violent pain in the bowels preceded the purging, which was attended with a very great proftration of ftrength, a wildnefs of the countenance, and the utmoft defpondency. And though it was not near fo *epidemical* as the Jamaica one, it was more malignant, or as Sydenham * expreffes himfelf, " of a more fpirituous nature."

In the equator one we had only 24 men ill, of whom four died †, one on the 3d, one the one 6th, the 11th, and one the 14th day. In the other we had 72 men bad, including relapfes and mild cafes, of whom nine only died, befides the vomical cafe; four of them died at the hofpital, but on which days of their ficknefs I am uncertain. The earlieft that died on board was on the 9th, and he had an exceeding bad fever accompanying it; one died the 20th of a relapfe, one the 22d, one on the 23d, and one on the 33d day, who had frequent relapfes.

Thefe few were the only material circumftances wherein the two dyfenteries differed.

SECTION III.

Reflections on the Dyfentery.

OF all the difeafes which infeft a fhip's company, the Dyfentery, in my opinion, if not the moft fatal, is at leaft equally fo with any other, and by far the moft loathfome. The conftant doleful complaints from the violent gripes, tenefmus, and other pains; the noxious fetor continually about themfelves, as well as arifing from the neceffary buckets; not to mention how extremely difagreeable fuch objects muft be to the fight; in fpite of all the means which can be ufed to prevent them, are evils peculiar to it alone. Yet great as they are, indubitably they are very much increafed when the weather is fo bad as not to admit the lower deck ports to be up in large fhips, or, as fometimes muft be the cafe, the hatchways in fmall fhips to be unlayed; for the foul air then being much more confined about the fick, and where the well people ly, it is confequently drawn into the lungs again and again by refpiration, and foon becomes more foul and noxious, which renders it unfit for the falutary purpofes of both healthy and fick.

Let me obferve, by the bye, that the laft mentioned circumftance is perhaps a much greater agent in enfeebling the feamen, and depreffing their

fpirits

* See Swan's tranflation of his works, p. 156, par. 6.

† Two more of them died at Port Royal hofpital.

ſpirits during bad weather, and occaſioning ſickneſs amongſt them, than all the inclemency of the weather to which they are expoſed upon deck in their watches. It is very pleaſing to obſerve the immediate alteration which appears in their countenances when the ſhip is well waſhed and aired, and they have cleaned themſelves after bad weather; from being quite ſallow and dejected, they acquire a healthy look, and freſh ſpirits.

But the poor dyſenterick patients ſuffer more particularly then, becauſe they are ſo weak, that even in good weather they are unable to get on deck to enjoy a moment's freſh air.

I take it for granted, that as it is to be apprehended infection might be communicated to the reſt of the ſhip's company from ſuffering the fluxes to eaſe themſelves in the head where the common ſeats are fixed, they ought not to be ſuffered to go there upon any account, though they were able: and when they arrive at a convaleſcent ſtate, one ſide of the head ſhould be allotted for their uſe only, and the well people prohibited from going thereto, and enjoined to prevent the convaleſcents from going to the other ſide, under the pain of being puniſhed.

If cleanlineſs in the ſick births is always neceſſary in other diſeaſes, there ſeems to be yet a more indiſpenſible neceſſity for their being kept remarkably clean in the dyſentery, for the reaſons already mentioned. But nothing can be added to the method which is already laid down for that purpoſe by Dr. *Lind*, in his eſſay on the moſt effectual means of preſerving the health of ſeamen—An eſſay which alone would have done that eminent phyſician great honor without the addition of his other valuable writings

SECTION IV.

Obſervations on different Medicines.

BUT what renders an attack of the dyſentery on board of a ſhip the more diſtreſſing, is, there not being any certain method of curing it yet diſcovered.

The bark, from its known qualities, and ſalutary effects in various diſeaſes, ſeems of all other to be the moſt ſuitable medicine for curing the dyſentery, after evacuations have been adminiſtered; but I am ſorry to ſay, that in the manner which I made trial of it, I found it came far ſhort of my intention, or expectation. It is true, I did not give it in a recent caſe, after the firſt vomit and purge, becauſe I apprehended that ſo early an uſe of aſtringents were abſolutely improper, and would have increaſed the inflammation, inſtead of curing the diſeaſe. Though, had I fortunately taken notice of that paſſage in Doctor *Lind*'s treatiſe on hot climates, * where, in his Directions for curing

* See p. 276.

ing the flux he recommends a mixture of the bark with opium, after vomiting and purging the patient, I certainly would have given up my own prejudice againſt ſuch an early uſe of it, and made a fair trial thereof. However, I muſt acknowledge in its behalf, that I found it the beſt corroborant in the declenſion of the diſeaſe.

Ipecacoanha performed nothing in the cure of either of the dyſenteries, to entitle it to the character of a ſpecifick, and moſt probably for the reaſon which Sir John Pringle aſſigns. *

Rhubarb toaſted or untoaſted, ſo ſtrenuouſly recommended by the learned Huxham, † was very far from being of that efficacy which he found it.

Diaſcordium with opium, another favourite medicine of that great author ‡ in the dyſentery, was not more efficacious than the former; nor the theriaca either. Opium, which was the immortal Sydenham's § principal remedy in the cure of the dyſentery, was barely a palliative in either of the two which are under our immediate conſideration.

Terra Japonica, was of no real ſervice either. How proper ſoever the great Boerhaave's ** method of treating the inteſtines, in an inflamed ſtate, may be, in the beginning of a dyſentery, other medicines are certainly requiſite to compleat the cure. Beſides, the inconveniencies that attend the frequent uſe of fomentations and injections, ſo as to be of any real ſervice on board of a ſhip, eſpecially when many are bad, are inſuperable.

As to the ſemiruba or lign. campechen. I had neither of them on board to make a trial of.

Section V.

The Method in which the Dyſentery was treated.

I Did not judge it proper to let blood in either of the dyſenteries, except in a caſe of the Jamaica one, which commenced with a hæmorrhage at the noſe. As the patient had been no way reduced by any preceding illneſs, to occaſion that ſymptom, I thought it a warrantable indication for diminiſhing the general maſs a few ounces. In a few other mild caſes of the ſame dyſentery which occurred on our paſſage to England, when our latitude was pretty high, and the weather cool, I took away blood ſparingly, becauſe ſome particular ſymptoms, in the courſe of the diſeaſe, not in its beginning, ſeemed to require it. Theſe few caſes indeed, all recovered, tho I do not attribute that

Y y by

* See p. 261 of his obſervations on the diſeaſes of the army. † Vid. obſervationes de aere et morbis epidemicis, tom. II. pagin. 106. ‡ ibid. pagin. 100. § Swan's tranſlation, ſect. IV. chap. 3.
** Vid. aphoriſm. 966, & 976

by any means to their being bled, but entirely to the favourableness of the attack of the disease. For I am firmly of opinion, that blood-letting is as pernicious in the dysentery in hot climates, as in the remitting fever, and chiefly for similar reasons.

The cure thereof was always begun by administering the ipecacoan, as an emetick. In the Jamaica flux, I generally gave from ten to five and twenty grains of the powder at one dose. Tho' it always vomited the patient well, and frequently procured him a more copious stool or two, I found that it operated by stool much better, when I gave five or six grains of it every hour, and repeated that quantity three times, after Sir John Pringle's * method In his manner therefore, I generally prescribed it in the equator flux and in the mean time, thin gruel, barley water, chamomile tea, or water with a toast in it, was allowed to be drank plentifully. † At night I always gave an opiate from the first of their complaining, to ease the violent pains, and procure some rest.

If the patient complained in the morning, and the operation of the ipecacoan was over, I gave him the same day, from one to two scruples of rhubarb, in the Jamaica flux; very seldom toasted; and tho' Huxham in his account of the dysentery which raged at Plymouth, in 1743, and of the manner of his treating it, gives the preference of all purges to rhubarb in these expressive words, " omnium sane optimum est rhabarbarum, quod " exhibendum est sæpius (tostum id semper si ab Indiis venit orientalibus) " cum nucis moschatæ, aut cinnamomi pauxillo," ‡ I changed the rhubarb purge in the equator flux, for the sal. cath. amar. which I found acted more powerfully, and with greater ease to the patient. I therefore generally gave sal. cath. amar. ℥i. dissolved in half a pint of thin warm gruel, and gave one third, or fourth part thereof, every half or three quarters of an hour, until it was all taken; allowing thin demulcent drink to work them off; and in the evening I ordered an opiate. The one which I made use of, was either the solid opium, or the tinct. theb. But when the vomit was taken in the afternoon, the purge was not administered until next day.

If the gripes were much relieved by the vomit and purge, and the flux was abated, the day after, whether it was the second or third of his complaining, I refrained from giving any other medicine than the opiate morning and evening, and allowed them demulcent drink at pleasure. § If on the contrary, the gripes continued violent, the stools small and frequent, and the patient had often an ineffectual desire of going to stool, I repeated the purge daily,

* See the place of his observations already cited. † Huxham, besides many others, recommend water. Vid. Loc. citat. ‡ Vid. ibidem. § In this I imitated Sir John Pringle; see his observations on the dysentery.

daily, until theſe complaints were relieved, and the opiate, if not oftner, at leaſt regularly every night.

When my patients were ſufficiently purged, and the inflammatory ſymptoms thereby moderated, I endeavoured to reſtrain the flux with ſmall doſes of ipecacoan, and rhubarb, given three or four times a day, and opiates, or with the diaſcord. cum opio, made into a mixture; a ſpoonful or two of which was given every two, three, or four hours, and an opiate at night. ℞. Spec. e. ſcord. cum op. ʒii. aq, ſimp. ℥viii. ſyr. commum. fiat miſtura.

But notwithſtanding the patient ſeemed to be recovering, it too often happened, that an exacerbation of all the complaints came on, either from the diſeaſe having been only palliated, or more frequently, perhaps, from ſome irregularity of the patients, and neglect of the attendants, ſo that I was obliged to repeat again and again, both the ipecacoan and purges, after I had begun to reſtrain the flux.

When the diſeaſe was thus violent and protracted, it became neceſſary to uſe, beſides the remedies already mentioned, and the white decoction, opiates repeatedly, to alleviate the violent pain; emollient fomentations for the abdomen; and emollient and anodyne clyſters compoſed of the decoct. ſem. lin. vel ſolut. amylon. with more or leſs of the tinct. theb. and likewiſe to uſe aſtringent and antiſeptick clyſters, which were made of the decoct. cort. peruv. et eleuther. vel flor. balauſt. cum opio, as well as to give aſtringents internally with wine: Theſe were the terra japonica, the cort. peruv. pulv. the decoct. cort. peruv. et eleuther. together with opium; but at beſt, they all proved too often ineffectual. However, to illuſtrate what I have ſaid upon this head, I ſhall add a number of the caſes of both fluxes.

SECTION VI.

Caſes of the Dyſentery which happened at Jamaica

CASE I.

WILLIAM Hutchins, marine, aged about 30, who never had been in a hot climate before, p. m. of June 10th, 1773, complained of having a flux upon him, and that he was violently griped at times. His ſtools were watery, his ſkin was drier and hotter, and his pulſe quicker than natural, and he was very thirſty. I ordered him an emetick of the ipecacoan, half a grain of opium at night, and plenty of thin gruel, or barley water for drink.

2d day. He found no alteration of his complaints. I preſcribed half a drachm of rhubarb, his drink and opiate at night, The rhubarb did not operate

operate well. 3d. He had a bad night, his ſtools were ſmall, frequent and bloody; his gripes were violent at times acroſs the abdomen, at others fixed in a point thereof, and the teneſmus was very troubleſome. I gave him pulv. rad. rhei. ℈ii. nuc. moſch gr. x. and his drink and opiate.

4th. He reſted better, and was eaſier, after having had ſome larger ſtools with his rhubarb. I preſcribed pulv. r. rhei gr. x. ipecacoan. gr. iii. m. f. pulv. to be repeated three times, and his drink and opiate as uſual, which gave him ſeveral pretty large ſtools.

5th. He was much better, p. m. the griping was more ſevere, and his ſtools frequent again. I ordered him four ſmall doſes of rhubarb and ipecacoan, and his opiate at night. 6th. He reſted well the firſt part of the night, and was better. I repeated his medicines. 7th. He continued much the ſame. There was always an exacerbation of his complaints p. m. I ordered half a drachm of rhubarb, and his opiate at night.

8th. He had a good night, was much better, and took his medicines as on the 5th, with decoct. alb. 9th. His griping when at ſtool, which was often, was very ſevere. I continued his medicines. 10th. He continued much the ſame, his pulſe was quick and ſmall, and his thirſt inſatiable. I repeated the purge and his opiate.

11th. He was rather better. I preſcribed pulv. ipecacoan. gr. vi. twice, which puked him, and gave him ſome ſtools, and his opiate at night. 12th. There was very little alteration on him, and he complained of a difficulty of breathing p. m. I ordered him the diaſcord mixture every three hours; the decoct. alb. and his opiate. 13th. He breathed eaſy, and his pulſe was pretty regular, tho' there was a wildneſs in his countenance, and his complaints continued; his ſtools were mucous, mixed with a little blood. I continued his medicines and decoction.

14th. There was no alteration made in his medicines, nor on him for the better. 15th, 16th. His flux ſtill continued, and he was much reduced. I preſcribed the following draught every four hours, and his opiate at night. ℞. pulv. cort. peruv. ℈i. tinct. cort. peruv. ʒſs. aq. ſimp. ℥iſs. ſacch. alb. q. ſ. pro hauſtus.

17th. He reſted very ill in the night, being very feveriſh the firſt part, and his ſtools were ſmall and frequent, together with his other complaints. I ordered him pulv. rhei. gr. xxxv. calomel, gr. ii. which purged him well, and his opiate at night

18th. He was very weak and thirſty, tho' in other reſpects much better. I preſcribed as on 15th and 16th. 19th. He continued better, was hungry and in good ſpirits. I repeated his medicines, and allowed him ſome weak mutton broth. P. m. his ſtools were frequent, and the gripes troubleſome.

20th,

20th. He was the ſame as on the preceding day. I continued his medicines, broth, and allowed a little wine; all of which agreed with him. 21ſt. He was recovering, and complained little. I ſtill ordered his bark, opiate and diet. 22d. As he lay in his hammock, a. m. after having ſtrained a good deal upon the bucket for a ſtool, an immoderate hæmorrhage, without pain proceeded ab ano, which increaſed upon the leaſt motion, and wet all his bedding before he knew of it. It could not be perceived upon examination from whence it proceeded; nor could it be ſtopped with tents dipped in ſtypticks, and introduced in ano, and opiates added to his draughts. I ordered an injection of a ſtrong decoction of balauſt. flor. with tinct. theb. to be adminiſtered, which entirely reſtrained it upon being repeated once; and when the injection returned, there was no blood mixed with it. The loſs of blood weakened him greatly, yet his appetite, which was in a manner voracious, continued. P. m. he was eaſy, and had no ſtool.

23d. He was very quiet all night, and had only one ſtool without any blood; his pulſe was thready and tremulous, and his countenance ghaſtly. I ordered his bark, wine, and diet to be continued. P. m. his extremities became cold; he was reſtleſs with his hands, picking himſelf and his bed clothes; had a hiccup, and died at 9 o'clock.

CASE II.

Michael Johnſton, ſeaman, aged about 48, complained the 18th of June of a flux, very ſevere griping, and pain in his bowels, which was ſometimes in one place of them, and then in another, exceeding violent. His ſtools were bloody. I ordered him an emetick, and an opiate at night, with demulcent drink.

2d. He was no better, and he had a ſevere pain in his loins. I preſcribed pulv. rhei. ʒſs. his opiate, and drink. P. m. his medicine did not purge him well. 3d. He was much the ſame. I repeated his rhubarb and opiate.

4th. He was yet no eaſier. I ordered him pulv. ipecacoan. gr. vi. three times, which purged and vomited him very well; and his drink and opiate.

5th. He was very uneaſy, his abdomen was ſwelled and tenſe, his ſtools were ſmall and frequent, and the teneſmus was violent. I ordered him pulv. rhei. gr. x. ipecacoan. gr. iii. f. pulv. three times (and the opiate at night) which purged him very little.

6th. His abdomen was leſs and ſoft, but his other complaints were the ſame. I preſcribed as on the fourth. 7th. He was much eaſier, and had leſs purging. I gave him farinaceous drink and his opiate only. P. m. he was feveriſh, and the ſwelling and tenſion of his abdomen returned. 8th.

He had no fever, and his abdomen was the ſame. I preſcribed as on the fourth.

9th. He had a tolerable night, after having been well purged with the ipecacoan. His abdomen was ſoft, and he complained of great weakneſs. I ordered him the diaſcord mixture. 10th. He was much better, tho' his flux continued. I repeated his mixture and opiate. 11th. There was no alteration until p. m. when the ſwelling and tenſion of his abdomen returned. I continued his mixture every three hours, the decoct. alb and opiate. 12th. He was much the ſame, and had ſevere gripes and pain about the bottom of his belly. I repeated the ipecacoan, as on the 4th, which operated chiefly downwards, and relieved him. After eating ſome broth, the ſwelling and tenſion returned.

13th. He was better, tho' very weak. I ordered him his mixture, drink and opiate. 14th. He complained of a ſickneſs, and pain at his ſtomach. I preſcribed pulv. ipecacoan. gr. x. and his opiate at night.

15th. He had the ſame complaints as on the 12th, and took the ipecacoan. gr. vi. three times, which brought away ſeveral ſcybala. 16th. He complained chiefly of a ſoreneſs in his bowels and weakneſs. I ordered him the mixture as before, and his opiate at night was gradually increaſed.

17th. He continued better, but had a pain in the left ſide of his abdomen. I repeated his mixture. 18th. He was troubled with flatulencies in his bowels, and expelled much wind per anum. He took his mixture as before.

19th, 20th, 21ſt. He was ſtill recovering, and continued his mixture. 22d. I ordered him a decoction of the cortex and eleuther. four times a day; his opiate at night, and allowed him wine, which he took regularly until the 26th, when he returned to duty.

This poor man relapſed, when we got to the northward, and the weather became cold, and was ſent to the hoſpital when we arrived in England.

CASE III.

Thomas Tileſly, marine, aged about 30, who came from Jamaica hoſpital a few days before, as cured of his flux, complained again the 19th of June, that his flux had returned on him the day after he left the hoſpital, his ſtools then were very frequent, he was ſeverely griped, and the teneſmus was quite painful. I ordered him an emetick, in two hours after pulv. rhei. ʒſs. demulcent drink, and an opiate at night.

2d. He was very little relieved. I preſcribed his rhubarb again, and the opiate at night. 3d. He had rather leſs pain, yet his ſtools were ſmall, frequent and ſlimy. I repeated his purge, drink, and opiate. 4th. He reſted

ill

ill from his purging, and a violent griping. I ordered pulv. ipecacoan. gr. vi. three times, and his opiate at night. 5th. He was much the ſame, and complained greatly of a ſuppreſſion of his urine, and a pain about the pubis, which he had for ſeveral days, although he did not let it be known. I preſcribed two ſpoonfuls of the diaſcord mixture every three hours, the white decoction, an emollient fomentation, and his opiate at night.

6th. He was much the ſame ſtill, and had his medicines and fomentation repeated. 7th. A. m. he complained of being griped. I preſcribed the bark as for Hutchins the 16th of his illneſs. 8th. He was very reſtleſs and hot in the night, from ſevere gripes, and ſmall frequent ſtools. I ordered the purge and calomel,* gr. ii. which operated well; and his opiate at night. 9th. He was very feveriſh and thirſty in the night, but his other complaints were eaſier. I repeated his bark and opiate as before. The ſuppreſſion of urine was gone.

10th. He had a frequent and ineffectual deſire of going to ſtool, and the teneſmus was troubleſome. I ordered his purge as on the 8th. P. m. as he was at ſtool, he puked a large lively round worm. 11th. He was much better. I preſcribed the bark and opiate.

12th. He was recovering, and repeated his medicines, with the white decoction and wine. 13th. He complained of ſickneſs at his ſtomach. I gave him pulv. ipecac. gr. x. which puked him, and afterwards repeated his bark, drink, and opiate.

14th. He was pretty eaſy, and continued his medicine regularly, until the 24th, when he returned to duty. He relapſed from the ſame cauſe as the preceding caſe, and was ſent to the hoſpital when we arrived, very much reduced.

C A S E IV.

Luke Coleby, ſeaman, a little inſane at times, aged about 44, complained the 21ſt of July, latitude at noon 31° 21″ of a flux, with which he had been ſeized two days before; his ſtools were then ſmall, watery and frequent, and attended with a very ſevere griping, and twiſting of his bowels. I ordered him pulv. ipecac. gr. vi. three times, which both pu ed and purged him well; and an opiate at night, with plenty of demulcent drink at pleaſure.

2d. He was no better, his bowels he ſaid, ſeemed to be cramped, or drawn into knots, and ſometimes as if they were cut acroſs the abdomen, or pierced

* Huxham preſcribed it, vid. pag. 100. tom. II. obſervat. de aere, &c. as alſo Sir J. Pringle and Cleghorn, to aſſiſt the rhubarb.

pierced with knives. I repeated his medicine as yeſterday, and the opiate twice. P. m. he was well purged again.

3d. He found himſelf much eaſier. I only ordered him his drink and opiate. 4th. He continued better. I preſcribed four ſmall doſes of rhubarb and ipecacoan, and his opiate with the white decoction.

5th. He complained of being very much griped and purged, and of the teneſmus. I repeated the ipecacoan, as on the firſt. 6th. He found himſelf very little eaſier. I ordered the powders as on the fourth. 7th. There was very little alteration, and he continued his medicines.

8th. His abdomen was very ſore, and he was much dejected. I repeated his medicines and drink. P. m. he had always an exacerbation more or leſs.

9th. All his complaints were more troubleſome. The diaſcord mixture was repeated every two hours, and the opiate morning and evening. 10th. He was eaſier, tho' much dejected. I continued his mixture, decoction, and opiates, and allowed him a little red port. 11th. He continued better, after perſpiring greatly in the night, about the head and neck. His medicines and wine were adminiſtered.

12th, 13th, 14th, and 15th. He was recovering. I allowed him his wine, ordered him pulv cort. peruv. ℨſs. with a little wine, four times a day, and his opiate at night. 16th. He was eaſy, unleſs when at ſtool, the griping was then violent, and the teneſmus very troubleſome—eſpecially p. m. I preſcribed a doſe of rhubarb, his bark and wine afterwards, and his opiate at night.

17th, 18th, 19th, 20th, 21ſt, and 22d. He could hardly be ſaid to have recovered any thing. He was weak, very much dejected, and there was always an exacerbation of the complaints and fever towards night. 22d. He complained that his ſtools which were mucous, were extremely hot. Flour boiled thin with water, to which a little wine, ſugar and cinnamon were added, was the only diet he would take, and that he ſoon purged after eating it. I repeated his bark and wine four times a day, and his opiate as before.

23d. He was much the ſame. I ordered him a doſe of rhubarb, and his opiate at night. 24th. There was no alteration. His diet, drink, and opiates only were preſcribed. P. m. he was ſeized with rigours.

25th. He had a tolerable night. I gave him four ſmall doſes of the ipecacoan and rhubarb. 26th. He continued better. I preſcribed an ounce and a half of a wine infuſion of the bark, four times a day, with his opiate and drink as before. P. m. his rigours returned with a fever.

27th. He reſted pretty well in the night. I ordered him pulv cort. peruv. ℨſs. tinct. cort. peruv. vin ℥ſs. aq. ſimp. ℥i. every two hours, beſides his diet, wine and opiate. I perſiſted in theſe medicines until the 36th day of his complaining, when I ſent him very weak and emaciated to the hoſpital, without

without the flux being quite gone. He was very untoward, thinly clothed, and frequently lay on the deck, in the courfe of his illnefs.

CASE V.

Rich. Enoch, marine, aged about 33, was feized the 29th of July 1773, with a chillinefs, rigours, and ficknefs at ftomach, which were fucceeded by a fever, headach, thirft, flux, and fevere gripes. He complained the 30th latitude at noon 41° 20″, and had a dofe of falts. I was not made acquainted therewith, nor faw him before the 31ft. His pulfe was then quick and rather foft; his fkin was dry and hot, his head ached very much, he was fick at ftomach, very thirfty, frequently purged, violently griped, and the tenefmus was very painful. I ordered him the ipecacoan to puke him, which operated well. P. m. his complaints were not relieved, and his tongue in the middle was brown and rough, with a red edge. I ordered a draught of the fp. minder. eff. antimon. and tinct. theb. fweetened with fugar, and plenty of acidulated drink.

4th Day of his illnefs. He refted very ill from his flux and griping, and perfpired very little in the night; the fever and fymptoms were more moderate a. m. tho' the flux and gripes were not relieved. His ftools were mucous ftreaked with blood, his countenance was bloated, and rather wild, and he complained of his toes being cramped. I prefcribed pulv rhei. gr. xxxv, which purged him well. P. m. there was an exacerbation of his fever, and his draught was repeated at night.

5th. He paffed a bad night. His pulfe was flower, his countenance was flufhed; he talked incoherently, he was fick at his ftomach, and the flux with its fymptoms was very troublefome. I gave him pulv. ipecac. gr. vi, three times; and though it operated well both by vomit and ftool, he was fcarcely at all relieved. I repeated his draught with more tinct. theb. and his acidulated drink.

6th. He refted the firft part of the night, he was purged very often, and violently griped afterwards. He was very fractious, his countenance was fallen, and he found himfelf much hotter, more thirfty and reftlefs at uncertain times, or now and then. I ordered a drachm of the cortex in a little red wine every two hours, and an opiate morning and evening. P. m. his flux continued, he had a hiccup, but was fubject to it; he drank fome coffee that his mefs-mates gave him; at 7 he had a perfpiration on him, and feemed better. His medicines agreed with him.

7th. He complained lefs, after having been eafy and little purged in the night. His pulfe was quick and fmall, he was extremely weak, his tongue

 was

was red, and he had a ſtupor on him. I ordered his bark with wine, to be repeated every hour. P. m. he ſeemed to be more ſtupid; his purging continued; he complained of no pain, he was very reſtleſs, and cried for air, and water to drink. I omitted his opiates morning and evening, and added tinct. theb. gt. v, to every doſe of his bark.

8th. He had only one ſtool in the night, he complained of no pain, his countenance was ſtill wild, he was unmanageable and delirious. P. m. he ſwooned away twice in the day, when he got out of bed to get to the bucket, and was worſe. I applied a large bliſter between his ſhoulders a. m. ordered him eight grains of camphor every four hours, and continued his bark with wine only every two hours, without the tinct. theb. and allowed him wine and water with a toaſt, for drink.

9th. He ſlept little from inquietude. He muttered, and complained of his bliſter, and his pulſe was ſmall and irregular. A. m. I ordered him camphor, gr. x, and the wine to be continued. There was a cadaverous ſmell about him p. m. and he had the hippocratick countenance. 5 p. m. I preſcribed moſch. gr. x. in a draught, applied bliſters to his ankles, and continued his drink. At 10 o'clock the hiccup was very troubleſome; he had convulſive rigours on him at times, and his reſpiration was laborious. I repeated his draught with twelve grains of the muſk, and ſupplied him with his drink.

10th. His medicines were ineffectual, and he continued growing weaker until 3 a. m. when he expired. Calculating the time properly, he died on the 9th day. From the prodigious fetor about him, he had certainly voided putrid, involuntary ſtools in his bed before his death; and that circumſtance prevented me from looking at his body before or after it; tho' I think it more than probable that there were external marks of putrefaction on it.

CASE VI.

Daniel Bingham, ſeaman, aged about 43, had been very ill of the dyſentery, for which he was ſent to Port Royal hoſpital, and returned uncured; but by taking medicine for ſome time, he recovered. However, he relapſed ſoon after, and was bad a fortnight before I learned that any thing ailed him. When I ſaw him on Auguſt 8th, 1773, latitude obſerved 45° 35″ he had a ſhocking appearance; he was extremely weak, quite ſallow, much bloated, the ſwelling was emphyſematous, his voice was weak and hoarſe, his throat was ſore, he was very often purged, violently griped, thirſty, had no appetite, was quite languid and deſponding, and his pulſe very feeble. As it was then late p. m. I only ordered him an anodyne and drink.

2d

2d Day of my ſeeing him, beſides his other complaints, he had a ſickneſs at ſtomach, and a teneſmus. I preſcribed pulv. ipecac. gr. vi twice, and camomile tea to drink. He was both vomited and purged, and had ſome eaſe. I allowed him a little wine, repeated his opiate at night, and applied an epithem to his throat.

3d. He had a bad night from his purging. I gave him pul. rhei. ʒſs. nuc. moſch. gr. x, continued his wine, repeated his opiate, and renewed his epithem.

4th. He was very reſtleſs, and complained much the firſt part of the night, yet was eaſier a. m. though none of his complaints were removed. I ordered him pulv. rhei. gr. vi. tart. emet. gr. ſſ theriac. androm. gr. v. aq. ſimp. ℥i. ſacch. alb. q. ſ. pro hauſta, four times a day; his wine and opiate at night.

5th. The flux and gripes were violent the firſt part of the night; he had no perſpiration on him, and he was weaker. I continued his draughts, wine and opiate. 6th. There was no alteration on him in any reſpect for the better, nor was there any made in his preſcriptions.

7th. He was eaſier than uſual the firſt part of the night; he got out of bed inſenſibly the latter, and had much pain in the abdomen. A. m. he ſlept ſome; when he awoke his tongue was black, his teeth were cruſted over with ſordes, and he was very thirſty. His pulſe was now extremely weak and irregular; and as the emphyſematous ſwelling was almoſt gone, he was quite ematiated. I applied a bliſter to his back a. m. and endeavoured to ſupport him with wine. He died at 6 p. m.

Query. Was this caſe what is termed, a ſcorbutick dyſentery?

I cannot properly inſert the caſes of the other two men who died of the Jamaica dyſentery, becauſe they were a conſiderable time at the hoſpital, whence they returned very ill, and continued ſo until they died. They both died with the ſymptoms of a putrid rectum. viz. vomitings, a ſuppreſſion of urine, and black putrid and very fetid ſtools. They took bark, were allowed red port, had opiates, emollient fomentations, and antiſeptick injections, with a light diet.

SECTION VII.

Caſes of the Dyſentery which happened to the ſouthward of the Equator.

CASE I.

THomas Watts, marine, aged about 32, who never had been in a hot climate before, was ſeized March 31ſt, 1774, p. m. with a flux, and complained

plained April 1ſt, lat. 00° 49″ ſouth, of a bloody flux, with violent gripes and pains in his bowels; he was ſick at his ſtomach, thirſty, and his pulſe quicker than natural. I preſcribed pulv. ipecacoan, gr. v. three times, which operated well by vomit; an opiate at night, and plenty of drink.

2d. He had a very bad night with his flux and gripes. His bowels were as if contracted into knots; and the teneſmus was exceeding painful. I preſcribed pulv. rhei, ℈ii. fomented the abdomen, and repeated his opiate at night with demulcent drink.

3d. His complaints were ſtill violent, his pulſe too was quick, and his thirſt inſatiable. I ordered him a doſe of ſal. cath. amar. and his opiate at night. P. m. he was well purged. 4th. He was eaſier in the night, unleſs when at ſtool, which was often, and then he was violenty griped. A. m. he complained of his bowels being very ſore. I repeated his purge, opiate and drink.

5th. He reſted tolerably, was much eaſier, and had a moderate perſpiration on him. I gave him only plenty of demulcent drink, and his opiate at night. P. m. he eat ſome mutton broth without my knowledge.

6th. He was often purged, ſeverely griped, and the teneſmus was very troubleſome in the night. I repeated the ſolution of the ſal. cath. amar. in a ſmall quantity every half hour, which procured him ſome large ſtools, wherein were ſcybala, and relied him greatly, and his opiate at night.

7th. He was frequently purged and weak, but was much eaſier, had a little appetite; and eruptions broke out on the left ſide of his check and chin. I ordered him four ſmall doſes of rhubarb and ipecacoan; a very light diet, and his opiate as before. P. m. he purged as ſoon as he eat any thing.

8th. The flux continued though he was eaſy, and perſpired freely. I repeated his powders, regimen and opiate, which was tinct. theb. gt. xl.

9th. He had an eaſy night, perſpired, and was hungry. I made no change in his preſcriptions. P. m. he made frequent vain attempts for a ſtool.

10th. His flux and the teneſmus continued, and the eruptions about his mouth looked angry. I ordered him the diaſcord mixture every two hours, with his diet and opiate at night. 11th, 12th. He was conſiderably better, and took his medicines.

13th. He was often purged in the night, and his bowels, he ſaid, were drawn together. I ordered the ſal. cath. amar. as on the 6th, and his opiate as uſual. He was not ſufficiently abſtemious. 14th and 15th. He was very weak, though much better. I repeated the diaſcord mixture and opiate, with his regimen as before.

16th. He was reſtleſs and much frightened the firſt part of the night, from a man's dying by him. I therefore repeated his opiate with a little wine. A. m. he was better, and took his medicine as before.

17th

17th and 18th. He recovered ſlowly, and no alteration was made in his preſcriptions. 19th. He had ſeveral bloody ſtools in the night without gripes. I ordered him pulv. cort. peruv. ʒſs. every two hours, with a little red wine, and his opiate, which was opii gr. i. at night.

20th. His bark purged him. Tinct. theb. gt. viii. was added to every doſe. 21ſt. He had an indifferent night with his purging. I preſcribed two ſcruples of the bark every two hours, with an opiate and wine, and the diaſcord mixture ſometimes, with a light diet. This method I followed regularly until the 27th, and then he could not be ſaid to have recovered in the leaſt. He was by no means abſtemious with regard to his diet, and whatever he eat, immediately paſſed through him. He was purged and griped. I ordered him pulv. rhei. gr. xii. ipecac. gr. v. theriac. androm. gr. viii. aq. ſimp. et ſyr. com. fiat hauſtus; it purged him well, and carried off the griping.

I again put him on his courſe of bark with wine and opiates, and a light diet, notwithſtanding which, he was very weak, and his flux continued on the 37th of his illneſs, when I ſent him aſhore to Antigua hoſpital.

C A S E II.

Daniel Marrow, marine, aged about 34, who never had been in a hot climate before, was ſeized the 1ſt of April, 1774, but did not complain until the 2d, lat. obſerved, 01° 16″ S. His ſymptoms were the ſame as the preceding caſes, and he was much dejected. I preſcribed the emetick, opiate and drink.

2d. He was violently purged and griped all night, his thirſt was inſatiable, and his pulſe was quick and full. I ordered him the purge of ſal. cath. amar. and though he was well purged, he found himſelf no eaſier; his drink and opiate were repeated.

3d. He was exceedingly troubled with inquietude in the night, from the violence of his complaints. A. m. he was a little eaſier, and had a perſpiration on him; yet his ſkin was nevertheleſs diſagreeably hot, and an uneaſy ſenſation remained on the fingers after feeling his pulſe. I repeated his purge and opiate as before, and indulged him with toaſt and water at pleaſure, as he was deſirous of it for his drink.

4th. He was eaſy while the effects of the opiate remained only; afterwards, he ſaid, his bowels were twiſted, drawn into knots, and ſeemed to be cut and pierced with knives; and his teneſmus was very painful. I repeated the purge and opiate, and continued his drink. P. m. he was eaſier after being well purged.

5th. He had a better night, was eaſier, and had larger ſtools. He was very weak, dejected; and a little thin ſago, which he requeſted and eat, did not agree with him. I gave him drink and his opiate only, beſides the ſago.

6th. His pain and teneſmus were eaſier, though he was very weak from inceſſant purging; and though ſago purged him, he was anxious for it. Inſtead of the diaſcord mixture which I ordered him, he was given three ſmall doſes of the ipecacoan, and his opiate at night.

7th. He was greatly fatigued in the night, with a frequent and fruitleſs attempt to eaſe himſelf; he was thirſty, much dejected, and his pulſe was quick and ſmall. I preſcribed pulv. rhei. ℈ii. theriac. androm. gr. viii. in a draught, and his opiate at night.

8th. He was much worſe; the fruitleſs attempt of eaſing himſelf continued, without any griping, he had an inordinate craving and anxiety, he lay on his face, his countenance was wild, his tongue was covered with a light brown mucous, and he wandered. Emollient clyſters † were injected, and the abdomen was fomented. I ordered the diaſcord mixture every two hours, the opiate to be repeated every four hours, allowed him red wine, and gave him the white decoction, or water and toaſt for drink.

9th. All his complaints were the ſame, and his ſtools were only a little ſanies, tho' he ſaid he was better—he now lay on his back, his medicines were continued. The injections were a ſtrong decoction of the cortex, and eleuther with opium. P. m. his fever increaſed, his tongue was black, his teeth were cruſted over with ſordes, his deſire of eaſing himſelf, with a pain again in the abdomen, and his other complaints, continued.

10th. He paſſed a very bad night, and grew worſe. His medicines were continued; a little warm wine was allowed him at intervals, and the antiſeptick injections were repeated. P. m. he had ſtill an ineffectual deſire to eaſe himſelf, he was extremely weak, his extremities were cold. At 8 o'clock, a hiccup came on, with convulſive catchings, and he died at midnight.

CASE III.

Daniel Waughan, marine, aged about 30, never had been in a hot climate before, was ſeized the evening of the 12th of April, 1774, latitude at noon, 04° 41″ S. the day that the preceding caſe was buried, with an excruciating pain in his bowels, which was ſoon followed by a flux. When he complained

† My mate informed me, that when he gave him the firſt injection, the anus was ſo much dilated, he could put all his fingers into it; that a bloody ſanies was dripping from it, and that ſcarce any of the injection was retained. He complained of great pain too in receiving them, and there ſeemed to be an obſtruction in it.

plained in the morning of the 13th, his flux and griping were very fevere, and he was exceffively dejected, and afraid of dying. I ordered him three fmall dofes of the ipecacoan, which vomited and purged him well, an opiate at night, and demulcent drink. P. m. he faid he was eafier.

2d. He continued eafier, but his defpondency and dejection were ftill the fame. I prefcribed a dofe of the fal. cath. amar. which purged him, and his opiate as before. P. m. he was feized twice with a deliquium. I allowed him wine now and then.

3d. He had a very bad night, from his having frequent bloody ftools, without pain or griping; he was very fick, and feized with his deliquium again a. m. His countenance was wild and frightened feemingly; he had fcarce any pulfe, and there was a cold clammy fweat over him. I ordered him cardiacks with wine, and applied a large blifter between his fhoulders. P. m. he was comatofe; he anfwered queftions very indiftinctly, and was very defirous of getting frequently out to ftool. His fkin became hotter a little before 9 o'clock, when he died. Fear alone feemed to have hurried him off fo quickly—He had been poxed, and, I underftood, took medicines of his own.

C A S E IV.

Benjamin Nixon, feaman, aged about 39, a hard drinker, on the evening of the 16th of April, latitude at m. 03° 04″ S. complained of a flux, fevere gripes, a vomiting at times, and great thirft; his pulfe was quick, and his fkin hot. I ordered the ipecacoan in fmall quantities, an opiate at night, and plenty of drink. P. m. the ipecacoan brought much bile up, and purged him a little.

2d. He had a very reftlefs night, and was no eafier. I prefcribed the falts, thin gruel, an opiate at night, and the white decoction. He was very thirfty p. m. and he had frequent fmall flimy ftools, yet was lefs griped.

3d. He found himfelf no better after much inquietude in the night. I repeated his purge, drink, and opiate as before. P. m. he faid his bowels were contracted to one place; his griping was violent, and the flux continued with a painful tenefmus.

4th. He was no eafier, but was very weak and much dejected. I ordered him a grain of opium every four or fix hours, as the pain required, fomented the abdomen, and gave him the common emulfion, and white decoction for his drink. P. m. his thirft was lefs, and he found himfelf a little eafier.

5th. He was much better. I repeated the opiates and his drink only. P. m. he had the violent gripes feldom, and though his ftools were frequent, they were larger, and voided with lefs pain.

6th.

6th. He found himſelf worſe. I preſcribed three ſmall doſes of ipecacoan, which vomited him a little, and purged him well, and his opiate at night. P. m. he was much eaſier.

7th. He reſted tolerably until midnight, when his griping began to be violent at times. I repeated his opiate twice, and continued his drink. P. m. he was not griped, but was very weak. 8th. There was hardly any alteration on him. I ordered the diaſcord mixture every two hours, his drink and opiate.

9th. He was better, tho' very weak. He got pulv. rhei. gr. xii. ipecacoan, gr. i. theriac. androm. gr. viii. in a draught, and repeated three times, inſtead of the mixture which I preſcribed. P. m. he did not find himſelf worſe.

10th. He had a cold ſweat on his face at times, tho' his complaints were eaſier, and his ſpirits were tolerable. I ordered the mixture, opiate twice, and his drink as before; and allowed him a little red port.

11th. He continued better, though very weak, and was diſturbed in the night with a man's dying; his ſpirits were good, and he had an appetite. I repeated his medicines, wine and drink. P. m. he complained of a little griping.

12th. P m. he became much worſe, he was ſeverely griped, and reached when at ſtool; he was much dejected, and his pulſe was quick and ſmall. His mixture, opiates and wine were given him regularly, and emollient clyſters with tinct. theb. injected.

13th. He had a bad night. A. m. he was eaſier, the reaching being gone. I ordered him the terra japonic. in the form of a mixture, with tinct. theb. aq cinnamom. ſp. ſyr. ſimp. et aq. commun. every two hours; his wine at intervals, and the antiſeptick and aſtringent clyſters to be adminiſtered. P. m. his ſtools became more frequent, his countenance hippocratick. the pain ceaſed, and a hiccup came on with extreme weakneſs.

14th. The hiccup increaſed. I repeated the medicines and his wine frequently. P. m. he ſpoke little, was extremely reſtleſs, and had a large putrid ſtool. The injections were continued, and a muſk draught given him every four hours. 15th. He was ſpeechleſs, yet took his medicines until 8 p. m. when he died.

CASE V.

Dudley Blackey, ſeaman, aged about 28, on the 19th of April 1774, lat. at m. 01° 05″ S. complained that he had had a purging for two months before; whether that was true or not, he was much emaciated, very giddy, his eyes were painful, he was then much griped when at ſtool, and his pulſe was

was ſmall and quick. I ordered him pulv. ipecac. gr. v. three times, an opiate at night, and demulcent drink.

2d day of his complaining. His flux, gripes, and the teneſmus, were very troubleſome. I preſcribed the ſal. cath. amar. ℥i. and his opiate. P. m. he was much better, having been well purged. 3d. He was much the ſame. I gave demulcent drink and the opiate only

4th. His complaints and purging were more troubleſome. I repeated the ipecacoan, as on the 1ſt, which vomited him a little, purged him very well, and relieved him much. He took his opiate at night.

5th. He continued better. I ordered him four ſmall doſes of rhubarb and ipecacoan, with opiates, and the white decoction. 6th. He complained of great weakneſs and hectick heats, and of being more purged and griped. I repeated his powders, opiates and decoction.

7th. He found himſelf no better, his giddineſs and other complaints being ſtill troubleſome. I ordered him the diaſcord mixture every two hours, and his opiate at night. P. m. he reached. 8th. He was much the ſame, and complained of a pain in the lower and back part of his neck. His medicines and drink were repeated, and I allowed him a little wine.

9th. He was ſick at his ſtomach, and much griped. I ordered him three ſmall doſes of the ipecacoan, his opiate, wine, and drink. 10th. After midnight his flux, teneſmus, and gripes became more ſevere. I preſcribed pul. rhei. gr. xii. ipecacoan, gr. v. theriac androm. gr. x. in a draught, which procured ſeveral large ſtools with ſcybala, and eaſed him. At night he took his opiate.

11th. The abdomen was tenſe, and he was ſeverely griped at times. I repeated his medicines, wine and drink, as on the 8th. 12th. There was no alteration on him, nor any made in his preſcriptions.

13th. He was no better of his flux, the hectick heats were greater, and he had pains in different places. I ordered him pulv. cort. peruv. ℈ii. tinct. theb. gt. xv. every two hours, and his wine. 14th. His head ached, and he had wandering pains. P. m. he complained of a tinnitus aurium. His medicines and wine were regularly adminiſtered.

15th. His flux, teneſmus, and griping, were eaſier, tho' his other complaints were more troubleſome. I preſcribed pulv. rhei. gr. x, tart. emet. gr. ſſ. theriac. gr. vi. three times, and afterward his bark and wine as before. P. m. his fever, wandering pains, and tinnitus aurium continued.

16th and 17th. He did not recover, though his bark and wine were regularly given him, and the rhubarb, with tart. emet. at intervals. 18th. He was ſent aſhore to Antigua hoſpital.

 CASE

C A S E VI.

Richard Hardie, marine, aged about 28, who had never been in a hot climate before, complained that he had been ſeized the preceding day, with a flux and griping, that his ſtools were more frequent, ſmaller, and bloody; his gripes and twiſting of his bowels were more violent. He had a painful teneſmus, and his thirſt was great, his pulſe was quick, and rather fuller than natural. I ordered three ſmall doſes of ipecacoan, demulcent drink, and an opiate at night. P. m. though he was well vomited and purged, he was not relieved.

2d. He had a bad night, and his complaints were the ſame. I preſcribed the ſal. cath. amar. his drink and opiate. 3d. He was not in the leaſt better, after a reſtleſs night. I repeated his purge with an opiate, his drink as before, and his opiate at night. P. m. he continued the ſame, and looked wild.

4th. He reſted a little in the night, and was not relieved by it. I repeated the three ſmall doſes of ipecacoan, and his opiate at night. P. m. his ſtools were very ſmall, frequent, and bloody; he reached at times; his hands were wet and cold, though his feet were warm; his countenance was wilder, and he wandered. I allowed him wine now and then, and repeated his opiate at night.

5th. He was very reſtleſs, and wandered more in the night. He had frequent ſmall ſtools, yet complained of no pains; and his legs were cold. I continued his wine, applied a large bliſter between his ſhoulders, and adminiſtered antiſeptick clyſters. P. m. the purging was abated, and his extremities were warm, but his wandering continued. I was informed that he fell down the fore cockpit hatchway in the night, when he was out at ſtool, through the careleſſneſs of the attendant—he complained of no part being hurt. At 8 o'clock he was very delirious, calling out for his companion who died the 1[illegible]th of the month, and died at midnight.

The reaſon why I have taken ſo little notice of the daily appearance of the ſtools, is, there being but few neceſſary buckets in the ſick births, and a number of the ſick uſing one, it rendered it impoſſible to diſtinguiſh the different ſtools; nor was it practicable to get a ſeparate bucket for every patient to remedy that inconvenience.

S E C T I O N VIII.—— *The Concluſion.*

IN the general account of the fever, as well as in the caſes which are inſerted to illuſtrate that, I have been particularly attentive to inſert the real

real occurrences only, and in the fame order which they appeared. I made it my principal ftudy to attend to the commencement of the paroxyfms and remiffions; and alfo to the different fymptoms of each. As to my manner of adminiftering the bark, I imitated no individual, for I never met with any author on the fubject who prefcribed it near fo liberally; nor does the fuccefs with which it was accompanied, give me the leaft reafon to repent of my having deviated fo widely in that particular, from men of the greateft eminence in the profeffion.

The daily fymptoms of the dyfentery are minuted exactly, together with the medicines which I prefcribed; from whence it is obvious, that I imitated Huxham and Sir John Pringle's method of treating it, but chiefly the latter, except in giving the bark when it became chronical; and I am forry to fay, that it was of very little fervice in the way which I gave it; nor can I help thinking that I was unfuccefsful in my method of treating that difeafe.

Many circumftances concerning the fever and dyfentery in particular, and the other difeafes in general which are mentioned in the Monthly Reviews, efcaped my obfervation perhaps, notwithftanding all my attention. However, I am hopeful that thofe which I did collect, and have faithfully reprefented, may not prove altogether ufelefs hereafter, to fuch of my Brethren as have never yet been employed on the coaft of Africa.

Indeed, as it is evident from the juft comparifon that I have made, page 15th, between the remitting fever, which was epidemick at different times on the ifland of Minorca, while *Cleghorn* was there; and the one which occurred on board of the Weafel (or even the Rainbow) on the coaft of Africa in the rainy feafon, that they differ only in a very few immaterial circumftances; notwithftanding, while the fever raged on board of his Majefty's fhips the Weafel and the Rainbow, they were failing at fo great a diftance from the land, that the noxious exhalations emitted therefrom, could not poffibly have any influence or effect upon the fituation of the fick.

And as I am convinced from my own obfervation on the difeafes which occur in the Weft Indies, and at Penfacola, and likewife from confulting moft of the authors who have wrote upon difeafes of hot climates, that thofe difeafes are effentially the fame in all of them, how widely foever they may apparently differ amongft the patients, from their peculiar habits, and external circumftances, nay, not any two cafes of all my patients, either in the fever or flux, were in every refpect alike. It can hardly be expected then, that one fever on board of a fhip in the Ganges, and another fever on board of a fhip in the river Gambia, in any feafon of the year, fhould be exactly fimilar, though the fever in both the fhips is of the fame genus, and will in like manner be cured by one and the fame method—bark alone. From thofe circumftances,

I have

I have ſufficient reaſon to think that this Journal will prove in ſome degree ſerviceable to thoſe of my Brethren who never yet have been in any hot climate, when their buſineſs calls them there—Should it fortunately anſwer that end, I ſhall think myſelf ſufficiently rewarded for my trouble in keeping it, and preſenting it with all ſubmiſſion to the Publick.

END OF THE JOURNAL.

POSTSCRIPT.

SECTION I.

Obſervations on Bark being uſed as a Preventive from Sickneſs on the Coaſt of Africa.

FROM the preceding Journal, it appears that the remitting fever was never epidemical on board of his Majeſty's ſhip Rainbow, but on the firſt voyage; and that they only were ſeized with it then, one caſe excepted, who had been employed on ſhore duty, and of whom very few eſcaped being more or leſs ill. But in what manner the noxious exhalations which are emitted from ſwamps, covered with impenetrable woods and ſhrubs, which contain putrid vegetables, corrupted fiſh and inſects, together with the aſſiſtance of heavy dews—operate upon the human body to produce fevers, only bare conjectures can be formed. To know that *arcanum*, would certainly be matter of great ſatisfaction to the curious, though perhaps the knowledge thereof could import far leſs advantage to us, than would the diſcovery of a method to prevent the poiſonous qualities of ſuch exhalations, from injuring thoſe people who muſt neceſſarily be expoſed to them, as the companies of his Majeſty's ſhips employed on the unhealthy coaſt of Africa, are. A diſcovery of that nature is perhaps thought too trivial to merit general attention; but it is of no leſs conſequence to his Majeſty's ſervice, than the preſervation of ſeamen's lives; the loſs of which, whatever may be ſuppoſed to the contrary, or how indifferently ſoever it may be eſteemed, is certainly a real national loſs; and therefore, whoever heartily endeavours to prevent it, merits the regard of the Publick.

Dr. *Lind* is the only perſon, who can be ſaid to have laboured ſtrenuouſly or ſucceſsfully in the prophylactick part of medicine, for the benefit of his

his Majeſty's navy in particular. His eſſay on the moſt effectual means of preſerving the health of ſeamen, and his treatiſe on the diſeaſes which are incident to Europeans in hot climates, were wrote principally for that purpoſe, though too little regard is paid to the excellent inſtructions which they contain, both by ſurgeons and others. For notwithſtanding that he has ſo highly condemned the dangerous practice of ſuffering the men to ſleep aſhore from their ſhips, on the dangerous or very ſickly parts of the coaſt of Africa, and even though the fatal effects of that cuſtom are woefully experienced on board of his Majeſty's ſhips, it is not yet exploded.

Without ſuffering the men to ly aſhore, they will be in too great danger of ſickneſs from doing their duty there by day; and as very little time is taken up in landing them every morning, and getting them on board again in the evening, the ſervice will thereby, ſtrictly ſpeaking, be more forwarded, inſtead of being retarded; becauſe the dangers to which their health is expoſed, chiefly from ſleeping aſhore in the night, will then be certainly avoided.

The ſituation of our watering party at Sierra Leon, the firſt voyage, and the weather, together with the ſituation of our people the night that they lay aſhore at St. Thomas's, ſoon after, are particularly taken notice of in the Journal. What an abominable place is the iſland of St. Thomas, for men to ly aſhore at, if there be a poſſibility of preventing it, when out of fifty and odd men, that were only aſhore one night, in a houſe with ſeveral large fires, few of them eſcaped without ſickneſs! Apprehending the conſequence that would enſue therefrom, and imagining that a large doſe of the tincture of bark might at leaſt be comfortable to them, I ſent next morning a ſufficient quantity of Huxham's tincture for each of them, which was carefully diſtributed by my mate, in a glaſs of wine that Captain Collingwood allowed them. No perſon by the bye could have expreſſed more uneaſineſs for their ſituation than he did, although it was not in his power to have prevented it. When they came on board, many of them were exceedingly dejected, and complained, but they were unanimouſly of opinion, that the tincture of bark and wine had been of very great ſervice to them.

Reflecting therefore on that circumſtance, I thought that a doſe of a ſtrong wine tincture of the bark, given to the men every morning, before they were to be ſent aſhore on duty upon the coaſt of Africa, might be very ſerviceable in preventing their getting fevers, I communicated to Captain Collingwood, the following voyage, my intention of proſecuting that ſcheme, if he approved of it; and would, in caſe there ſhould be a neceſſity, give orders for their taking the tincture. I intimated to him, at the ſame time, in what manner it might be introduced on board of his Majeſty's ſhips employed on that ſervice afterwards, through his aſſiſtance, if it ſucceeded in the Rainbow. He readily concurred with me to make a trial of it, and aſſured me if it did ſucceed,

 ceed,

ceed, that he would use his utmost endeavour to get such a salutary measure introduced on board of his Majesty's ships employed on that coast. I then commenced a correspondence* with him upon the subject; and he was pleased to direct Captain *Robertson*, commander of his Majesty's sloop Dispatch, by a letter, to advise Mr. *Perry*, the surgeon under his command, to adopt the same scheme, and at the end of the voyage to get his report of its effects in writing, and transmit it to him; which, together with my report of its effects on board of the Rainbow, he sent up to the Secretary of the Admiralty, as well as all the letters, and copies of letters which were wrote upon the subject, inclosed in one, wherein he recommended the scheme to their Lordships, and requested that they would be pleased to allow us for our expence in making the tincture, as soon as the ship arrived in England.

In their Lordships answer to Captain *Collingwood*, they were pleased to inform him, that they had sent the reports of the surgeons upon the subject to the Commissioners for Sick and Hurt, to know their opinion of it; and desired them to call upon the surgeons for their accounts of the expence which they had been at in making the tincture. The Sick and Hurt Board accordingly wrote to us separately; and in my answer to them, I inserted the formula of the tincture, which was ℔vi. cort. peruv in crass pulv. rad. gentian. incis. ℔ii. rad. serpent. cont. ℔i. put into a quarter cask of wine—but we sailed again for the coast, without my hearing any more from them. I therefore persisted in my own scheme, only adding cort. per. ℔i. a proportionable quantity of the rad. & aurant. parv. ℔ii. to the quarter cask of wine, the last voyage, more than I had done the preceding one: and when we returned to England, I gave Captain *Collingwood* a report of its effects, which he sent, with the different letters on the subject, and one of his own to the same purport as the one he had sent before to the Secretary of the Admiralty, who informed him by their Lordships' directions, that they had ordered the Commissioners for the Sick and Hurt to repay the surgeons their expences for making the tincture, and to send them their opinion of the matter But previous thereto, that board thought proper to consult the physicians of the different hospitals, and some of the most eminent physicians in town, thereon, who were unanimous in their opinion.—They afterwards acquainted their Lordships, that the happiest effects might be expected from giving the bark, as a preventive from sickness, to the men who might be sent ashore on duty upon the coast of Africa; but that instead of a tincture, they had recommended a drachm of the powder, with a gill of wine to be given every morning and evening.

In

* It continued afterwards, until the Rainbow arrived at Spithead from her last voyage.

In consequence of which, the lords of the Admiralty were pleased to orde bark and wine to be purchased at the Government's expence, and to be sent on board of his Majesty's ships the Pallas and Weasel, the two ships which were sent to the coast this year, with directions to the commander of the Pallas concerning it; and likewise ordered the Commissioners for Sick and Hurt, to send such directions to the respective surgeons, as they thought proper, with regard to administering them; and to direct them to keep a particular account of the effects thereof, and transmit the same to them when the ships returned to England. So that I have at last the pleasure of seeing that scheme, which in all probability will be the means of preserving many lives to his Majesty, established by their Lordships authority, through the assistance of Captain *Collingwood*, and the candour of the Commissioners for Sick and Hurt, who have since repaid me for my expences.

In discoursing with Dr. *Lind* on the matter upon our arrival in England, after I had first made trial of it, he informed me that he had for the like purpose recommended, in his Essay on the most effectual means of preserving the health of seamen, a bark bitter; and on my telling the Doctor that I never had seen that valuable essay, he showed me therein the article mentioned, and was so obliging, as to insist on my accepting of the copy of the Essay--which I acknowledge is not the only favour that he has conferred on me. I own too, that I was a good deal pleased to find, that I had adopted that proposition of the Doctor's, without knowing that it was one of his. Before I formed my scheme, I knew that the people on the coast of Africa, as well as the officers and gentlemen on board of his Majesty's ships, took a little tincture of the bark, either in a glass of wine or water every forenoon, as a stomachic; but I never heard of its being given to the ships' company as a preventative from sicknefs. Therefore, as I succeeded in perfecting it* by the method and assistance which I have mentioned, I hope it will prove an inducement to my brethren, for introducing improvements of greater moment on board of his Majesty's ships, for the health of the seamen; and I hope that my desire of propagating such an useful remedy, will plead an excuse for my having been so particular on the head. †

SECTION

* See the success with which it was attended, mentioned in the Monthly Review.

† N. B. An account of the success of the scheme, on board of the Pallas and Weasel, shall be sent to the Printer, when the Pallas arrives.

SECTION II.

Reasons offered for the necessity of supplying his Majesty's ships, employed on foreign service, with Bark, after the same manner that they are supplied with elixir of vitriol, or Doctor James's *Powders.*

PEruvian bark is essentially necessary in curing various diseases of all climates, particularly of hot ones,; the consumption thereby is so great, and the price thereof consequently so high, that the surgeons of his Majesty's navy not being able to purchase a sufficient quantity to serve the purposes for which it is really wanted on foreign service, lose many of their patients lives, which they could otherwise preserve.

I am sorry to say, that this was my case in 1769, upon the coast of Africa, in the Weasel, and that it was Mr. *Curry*'s likewise, surgeon of that same sloop, and upon the very same station, in 1774. Notwithstanding we had each of us more than thrice the quantity which is put up in the medicine chest for foreign service, it was not half sufficient for the number of patients we had. Mine were thirty-two bad cases of the remitting fever, besides a number of other cases wherein I did and would have prescribed the bark more freely; and upon a medium, every one of those thirty-two cases would have required ten ounces, which in all would have been 20 ℔. and bark at Apothecaries Hall, on a moderate calculation, is twelve shillings and sixpence per ℔. and was lately at the enormous price of seventeen shillings and eight-pence there; so that 20 ℔. would have stood me in twelve pounds ten shillings, above one fifth of my pay; and, at least, I might allow 4 ℔. more, for other uses, which in all, would have cost fifteen pounds, the fourth part nearly, of my annual pay, for one article of medicine only.

At the end of my Journal for that sloop, I represented to the Commissioners * for Sick and Hurt, the distress that I was in for want of bark, with the consequences which attended it; and entreated them that they might be pleased for the good of his Majesty's service, to use their endeavour to get all his Majesty's ships, employed in hot climates, supplied with it, after the manner that they are supplied with elixir of vitriol, or James's powders.

As I reeceived no answer from that board, I set on foot a plan for the surgeons petitioning the Admiralty, to allow bark for his Majesty's ships employed on foreign service, after either of the ways which I have mentioned, or as they should think proper; but unluckily, being ordered to sea before I could

* The predecessors of the present Commissioners, but they did not think proper to take the least notice of the matter.

could get it completed, the matter dropped in my abſence, and has not ſince been renewed.

I would therefore, with all deference, beg leave to recommend it to the moſt ſerious conſideration and attention of the preſent Commiſſioners for Sick and Hurt; the effecting of which, will not only be a taſk ſuitable to the known humanity of theſe Gentlemen, but will in like manner evidence their ſtudy to promote the real benefit of his Majeſty's ſervice in their department.

But it may be urged, that my plea for requeſting this expenſive innovation, is only grounded on two inſtances which occurred upon the coaſt of Africa; and that his Majeſty's ſhips employed there now, are furniſhed with means for preventing ſickneſs from ſhore duty, whereon the principal danger of contracting ſickneſs there depends I grant it. Yet the time of theſe ſhips, after they leave that coaſt, continuing in a hot climate, where the people are always liable to bad fevers and other ſickneſs, is very conſiderable; and that therefore, they ought to be better prepared againſt ſuch evils than the ſurgeons are capable from their circumſtances, to prepare themſelves.

Should this argument be deemed inſignificant, I beg leave to furniſh them with a far more fatal inſtance than either of the two which I have mentioned, of the want of bark in the army, as well as in a large fleet of his Majeſty's ſhips during the late war, *at the reduction of Havannah,* when thouſands, I may venture to affirm, were loſt for want of bark chiefly.—A period therefore, which, for the mortality both of ſeamen and ſoldiers, will be memorable throughout his Majeſty's dominions for many ages. There was a general want of that precious medicine, both in the fleet and the army, when they were very ſickly, until providentially, a capture of a large quantity thereof, was made in one of the enemies ſhips, which was carefully divided between the fleet and the army.

I ſhall now leave this important matter before the Sick and Hurt Board, for the Commiſſioners to reflect on as they think proper, after preſuming to ſay, that if they do procure his Majeſty's ſhips which are employed in hot climates, to be ſupplied with bark, after either of the ways which I ha. taken the liberty to mention, or as they themſelves think fit, at the Government's expence, it will be a certain method of preſerving annually to his Majeſty, many valuable lives, which otherwiſe will be loſt. No expence whatever, in my opinion, can juſtly be put in competition with the preſervation of the lives of his Majeſty's ſeamen or ſubjects.

I beg leave to acquaint my brethren, in the mean time, that Doctor *James Hoſſack,* Phyſician to the royal hoſpital at Greenwich, who ſurveys our medicine cheſts, and the liſts of ſupplies which we write to Apothecaries Hall for, is not only ſo obliging as to order double the quantity of bark to be put

 in

in our chefts, to what is fpecified in the old eftablifhed printed form of fupplies, and a proportionable lefs quantity of other articles of medicines, which are feldom wanted, but alfo indulges the furgeons with any medicines of their own, that they apply for, inftead of thofe mentioned in the printed invoice Though, unlefs they amount in value to the fum which is eftablifhed for us to lay out for medicines, according to the rate of the fhip we are in; they may expect, that he will order fuch an addition of other articles, which are moft fuitable for the ftation that the fhips are going upon, as will make up that fum.

By this means therefore, until we are fupplied with bark at the Government s expence, which I fincerely hope will be foon, they may provide themfelves with a greater quantity of bark, and of the other moft ufeful articles of medicine, in place of thofe which are lefs ufeful, without putting themfelves to any extraordinary expence, which many of them perhaps have done hitherto, from their not knowing this circumftance.

I muft alfo do Doctor *Hoffack* (whofe friendfhip I have been favoured with for fome years) the juftice to declare, that it was chiefly owing to his perfuafion, that my Journal and Obfervations would hereafter be ferviceable to Surgeons who have never yet been in a hot climate, particularly on the coaft of Africa, when they go there, that I was prevailed upon to offer them to the Publick.

Printed in the United States
By Bookmasters